Brain Fog

Eliminate Symptoms and Improve Memory

(Healing Pathways for Mental and Emotional Health Answers)

Phillip Pendleton

Published By **Bengion Cosalas**

Phillip Pendleton

All Rights Reserved

Brain Fog: Eliminate Symptoms and Improve Memory (Healing Pathways for Mental and Emotional Health Answers)

ISBN   978-0-9950956-1-8

No part of this guidebook shall be reproduced in any form without permission in writing from the publisher except in the case of brief quotations embodied in critical articles or reviews.

Legal & Disclaimer

The information contained in this book is not designed to replace or take the place of any form of medicine or professional medical advice. The information in this book has been provided for educational & entertainment purposes only.

The information contained in this book has been compiled from sources deemed reliable, and it is accurate to the best of the Author's knowledge; however, the Author cannot guarantee its accuracy and validity and cannot be held liable for any errors or omissions. Changes are periodically made to this book. You must consult your doctor or get professional medical advice before using any of the suggested remedies, techniques, or information in this book.

Upon using the information contained in this book, you agree to hold harmless the Author from and against any damages, costs, and expenses, including any legal fees potentially resulting from the application of any of the information provided by this guide. This disclaimer applies to any damages or injury caused by the use and application, whether directly or indirectly, of any advice or information presented, whether for breach of contract, tort, negligence, personal injury, criminal intent, or under any other cause of action.

You agree to accept all risks of using the information presented inside this book. You need to consult a professional medical practitioner in order to ensure you are both able and healthy enough to participate in this program.

Table Of Contents

Chapter 1: The Functions Of The Brain 1

Chapter 2: The Connections That Connect The Brain And Memories 23

Chapter 3: How To Keep Your Mind Sharp Throughout Your Life 34

Chapter 4: Brain-Healthy Foods To Increase Brain Power 41

Chapter 5: Aphasia (A Neurological Condition) 45

Chapter 6: Brain Fog 73

Chapter 7: Diet 83

Chapter 8: Physical Activity 95

Chapter 9: Guided Meditation 105

Chapter 10: First Thing You Require Is A Space To Be Seated 118

Chapter 11: Guided Visualization A Walk Through The Forest 150

Chapter 12: The Sky Of Your Mind 173

Chapter 1: The Functions Of The Brain

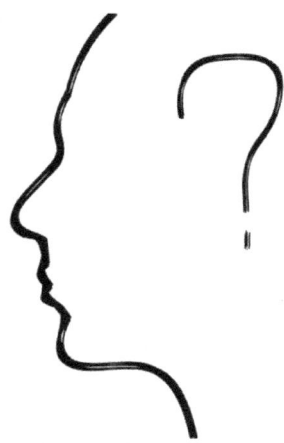

Do you have a problem with your mind or body? Does there exist a distinct distinction that can be drawn between the rules or principles and the relationships which govern those mental (body as well as the brain) as well as the mental (mind) elements of our being? This could mean that the mind operates independently of brain and body but this is not the reality. Is the mind independent from brain and body? Could the brain and the body exist in absence of the mind? The mind, on contrary, is not able to be existent without the body or the brain. What happens after you've killed the brain and body? It's unlikely that you're thinking about what your brain and body went, but your mind remains.

In contrast there is the possibility of having severe mental illness or brain injury which has left you disabled, however your brain and body could remain alive via life support. This technically keeps your body and brain alive. Though the brain and body remain in motion by artificial means but there isn't any consciousness that can be achieved. Although the body and brain do recover because of these amazing medical interventions however, the mind won't always be restored. What number of times has the life support system been shut off due to the fact that, although the body and brain can technically remain alive for an indefinite period of time but there's no assurance that the mind will be able to recover? It is possible to have a healthy and functioning mind does not depend on the body or brain and body, while the mind's existence is totally dependent on working body and brain. Mind is connected to the body, and is a service for the brain and body. The mind is not a an independent existence.

Brain and mind aren't identical. An example of how brain can exert control over your body's functions in areas that the mind is not able to control is through the autonomic nervous system. It ensures that the heart beats as well as your lung's lungs are breathing while your mind rests. The truth is that your thoughts are constantly wandering. Not solely while you sleep as well as in the event of a fallout due to reasons other than being a lack of oxygen. Your brain, on contrary, is constantly alert and in constant motion. Although your brain is totally awake, your brain can't direct your heart to slow down or tell the lungs to stop breathing.

The brain is not able to effectively argue against hunger, thirst or fatigue. In the end, your brain is the one in charge. The brain is able to continue to function and exist in the event that your mind remains in limbo yet the mind remains working when it is still in limbo. The absence of a brain is not the same as having the existence of a mind. However, no mind implies the absence of a brain. This should be evident!

Does the Mind Create the Brain?

It is straightforward to envision that a brain is not a mind and it's a bit more difficult to envision a mind without having a brain. The mind, the thoughts, feelings as well as emotions comprise the mind. Mind can be linked to consciousness as a whole and self-awareness specifically. Your mind, however, is stuck in Neverland even when you're asleep or drunk, numb or under anesthesia following surgery or sleeping. But it's hard to say that your brain was actually in Neverland when you were sleepy and drunk or intoxicated. Minds would perish when the brain is destroyed. However, like I've previously demonstrated mental incapacities do not mean that brain capacity is impaired. In the end, there is no doubt that the brain as well as the mind are interconnected to each other, and that the mind serves the brain.

The mind is formed by mind's electric (energy) as well as chemical (matter) activities. The term "brain dead" is used to describe as a complete cessation of brain electrically or chemically produced activities. When this happens one is believed to be dead biologically until artificial supply of chemicals as well as electricity are employed to maintain their body's functioning such as when they are in life support. If your brain has died the mind too is dead. If there were a non-physical part of mental activity your mind could be working in the brain that is dead.

What Is the Definition of Consciousness?

Evolution and natural selection has given consciousness a function or, at the very least, importance in terms for survival of the best. The term "consciousness" refers to the awareness. If you're asleep and aware, there is a good likelihood of not passing your DNA to your children because there's no awareness of what's happening within your. While consciousness could have developed in response to an accident however, the fact that consciousness exists now eliminates any need for metaphysical or philosophical language for expressing consciousness.

Consciousness develops based on awareness. There could be three distinct levels of consciousness. In the first place, you're conscious of the surroundings. It is possible to feel the wind and lightning strikes, feel the sound of thunder, smell and taste the food cooking. Another thing you're mindful of, or conscious about is the health of your physique. The nose is itchy while your heart is beating and you're suffering from acid reflux and are tired. When you're conscious of or aware of the internal functioning of your mind you also become aware of them.

The depression you feel is due to the dark, cold and wet winter days. You're devastated by the passing of your pet. You decide it's best to start cooking your dinner. When the sales for mid-season begin, you envision what you'll get for your money. Therefore, the center of your mind is comprised of three realities (environment as well as body as well as your thoughts) which require your attention and, in turn you are aware of them.

Are there any reasons to know? It's important to take this seriously! The simplest definition of consciousness is consciousness, which is the awareness of your body, the thoughts of one's and the world around us. In dealing the challenges life can throw at you, consciousness must be an integral part of the toolbox. When I say living, I don't only refer to people of today as well as all living things that have survived, but not flourished over the geological time.

The organism won't endure, much less flourish if it is not aware or understanding of its environment as well as internal processes. It is essential to be alert to any possible predators or prey in the immediate area. If you are hoping to transfer the genes you have, take note of the body's signals when you are mating. When your senses alert that you are in danger, then your body has to decide whether it is better to defend yourself or run away. Living organisms is awake and aware in order to be able to function. It is necessary to be conscious in order to live.

Are there any particular goals for our human brain? "Special purpose" or "special reason" suggests that our consciousness is directed or managed by some method. Natural selection could have led to a purpose however, the term "special" reason is superior to this notion. The awareness we have increases our odds of survival, which allows us to transmit our genes to the next generations. When we "live" as simulations in a universe that is simulated

Perhaps humans were created specifically to keep simulations running. The Supreme Programmer is our next step in creating more simulations in the same way that chickens produce many eggs.

Is awareness a delusion? If so it is unlikely that you'll be able to live long enough for success. The concept of consciousness is based on your awareness of your current state of your immediate environment and awareness of the condition of your body at the moment, and awareness of the state your mind is in. If the physical environment as well as your body appear to be illusions, I would guess that you're being a brain-in-a-vat since your state of mind is not an illusion "I believe that I am" I am convinced is the appropriate quote. Your actions are based on the information your mind (yourself) informs you about for example, if I'm constantly yawning; maybe I need to get some sleep and I hate my neighbour, and I'm walking next door to shoot the guy. In the end I interpret the adage that is famously known as "I react, and therefore are." If you consider (awareness) and respond to stimuli, it's highly unlikely you'll act or react stimulus that is not real (self-awareness). If the stimulus you are experiencing isn't an illusion and your awareness isn't affected, neither are you and your perception of it.

It is clear that in dealing with quantum physics it is necessary to deal with an apparent awareness (or awareness) which elementary particles seem to have so one can claim that consciousness was born in the early stages of Big Bang, I'll ignore this and just consider consciousness as a natural characteristic of living things and that's pretty much what is the general consensus. The terms consciousness and awareness are two terms that can be interchanged. Cells or any unicellular organism which emerged from any type primordial soup must be able to do it with its mind intact, or else it would not be able to be a part in the biochemical process that is a living organism. Life forms were required to begin eating other living types, or after the nutrients of the primordial soup became diminished, the struggle to survive of the most fit was evident at the start of time and even more or less.

The first animals with monocellular DNA had to comprehend that the basic soup had nutrition in it and others could be potential predators or prey. The creatures would have not lived and thrived in the absence of the knowledge or were aware. Therefore that it's no surprise that awareness and early living forms of life appeared virtually in the same time. It is essential to be aware for the survival of our species, as it was when the first species emerged.

The physical nature of consciousness is the only thing that matters. Being able to alter your consciousness when you eat physical substances can be proven by the pudding. Some of these substances are known as substances, both legal and legal. Similar to the way that certain foods can. In the event that you do not get enough oxygen, the degree of consciousness may change. Medical illness or injuries like those that cause amnesia can cause a loss of consciousness. The process of sleeping is an illustration of how the chemistry in your body including your brain, could affect the state of consciousness you are in. In order to create sleep it is necessary to administer an anesthetic that is a certain physical drug, could be given. When it is not in contact with people, it's impossible to say that a cat who took catnip has the same mindset the cat who isn't.

The Powers of the Subconscious

Sincerely I am of the opinion that our subconscious mind is a less understood part of the brain than conscious. I am awestruck by the things the subconscious can accomplish that is not limited to humans however, in all animal that even has the simplest essential neural network system elements.

The body will usually repair its own way. If you suffer from a bruise, scrape or muscle tear and bone fragment or even a headache your body is likely to heal itself. However, it'll become more difficult as you get older. Naturally, there will be instances when your body is not able to heal itself and, in these instances, specific medical (such in pharmaceuticals) or physical (such such as surgeries) treatment must be carried out externally. Sometimes, physical or pharmacological therapy is not efficient. After surgery, however the body's natural chemistry like blood clotting, the chemistry that is consumed by outside sources, or the manipulation of chemistry by the mind, are the primary factor in the healing process.

Chemistry and the mind have an interplay. The chemistry in the mind as well as the chemistry of the body can both influence the other. If everything else fails, will the mind win over material? Is it possible for the mind to help the body heal without the need for chemicals? Does it make sense for positive thoughts to have therapeutic effects without the requirement of the use of energy or matter? It is not likely There two main reasons why this is the case. Healing includes physical elements (such as medicines) that affect physical objects (like the body's tissues). Physical entities are not able to affect the physical objects. Another reason is that individuals lose their lives despite using all their mental power to stop the event from occurring. If you are diagnosed with cancer, it is incurable. It is not able to be treated with surgical procedures, prescription medicines, or the natural body chemistry. This cannot be altered by the power of imagination.

An attack on your heart that is serious causes your heartbeat to stop. The power of wishful thinking won't help you heal or re-start your heart, only a medical intervention could help you save time. If only the mind had the power to heal the body after everything was failing and there was an inexplicable reason why anyone should be dead. Every person who ever passed away has a brain and would use this mind in a mad endeavor to stop the death. It's not the way the mind works.

Awareness and consciousness are the same thing. This simply means that you're conscious of the world around you. All that is around you that you are able to observe with the five senses is as your surroundings. This could mean that you're aware of what your body is going through on an inner scale. It could be a sign of being conscious of your emotions, thoughts as well as other concerns. In the end, you're aware or even alert to the fact that your house is hot. Perhaps you're conscious or conscious of headache. It is possible that you are conscious of or even aware of the anxiety you feel regarding your car's running out of fuel. Being able to recognize and take action on the numerous parts of oneself which have been documented is called self-awareness.

Many people experience overheated are suffering from headaches, feel hot, or are in need of filling up their vehicle, self-awareness recognizes certain aspects of your experience which are specific to your situation. This awareness lets you deal directly with issues that occurred to you and, at minimum, address these issues when you're able. Not being able or willing to tackle another person's problems is a self-awareness issue on its own.

So, when you recognize that you're running hot then you switch on your air conditioner. When you realize that you're suffering from headaches, you choose to try a few aspirin. You decide to stop at the station to fill up your tank with gasoline is based on your realization the fact that your vehicle needs refueling. Self-awareness responds to what your conscious or awareness tells you.

What exactly are altered states of consciousness? Your brain's chemical chemistry represents the degree to which you are aware regardless of what that might be. There is evidence that suggests changes to the brain's chemistry that are caused by the practice of meditation sleep and illness or injury and also medications of all sorts that are present in food, can make your regular consciousness change however, sometimes by so little that it's not noticeable. The consciousness continuum includes different states of consciousness that can be described as different perspectives on the normal state of consciousness. There are many kinds of states of consciousness just like the different frequency bands of the electromagnetic spectrum that range from very small to extremely lengthy. What does the gamma-ray spectrum reveal about the regular visible spectrum, or radiation wavelength spectrum? All of them are the same yet they're distinct, but they're identical.

The wavelengths gradually become more pronounced from one particular label (gamma Ray) before moving to the following (visible) (radio). A state of mind that is altered blends with another one due to changes in the brain's chemical composition, suggesting that there isn't an unambiguously defined standard state of mind. However, every state of consciousness can be considered to be an altered state of mind over all other states. In spite of their distinct characteristics however, all states of consciousness have the same conceptual basis.

It is clear that having low sleep quality or getting sufficient sleep because of your work schedule can affect the way your brain functions after you have figured it out. You will be able to focus better by obtaining the seven to eight hours of quality sleep which experts suggest. Lack of sleep affects both your emotional and physical wellbeing. Actually, it impacts the overall health of your metabolism physical and mental performance, as well as your energy levels.

When you sleep all day, the whole experience will be recollected in your mind as well as reflected in your past memories. It is more likely for you to become forgetful when you don't get an adequate night's sleep. Concentration can be impaired. You'll have a trouble time understanding and remembering information.

In determining the amount of sleep is required to stay active and healthy it's difficult to provide an answer that is general in nature since the conditions vary from one individual and also from age to age category. Children, for instance, require sixteen hours sleep each day. Some people need 5-6 hours sleep in comparison to others who require between 10 and 12 hours of sleep generally, all require between 7-8 hours.

Pregnant women in early stages require greater sleep also.

Many people believe that only those with sleeping issues suffer from insomnia. However, there are many who have trouble falling asleep, before waking up early in the early morning. Yet, people who do not fall asleep right upon waking up will likely suffer from an sleeping disorder of a certain kind. People who aren't sleeping well this is the reason they sleep fast. Research suggests that a absence of sleep impacts memory and productivity. It is said that your ability to do things is reduced. This is why sleeping troubles affect how your brain operates.

Chapter 2: The Connections That Connect The Brain And Memories

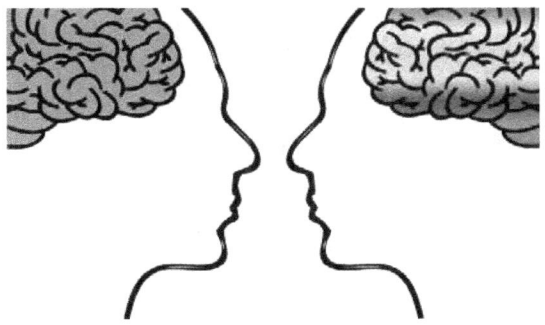

Each human action is psychomotor. It is the brain that is the primary control of all parts of human functioning. It is vital to live an active and healthy lifestyle if one is looking to lead a healthy and prosperous life. Many factors could influence how your mind develops in either a positive or negative way. Based on research it is believed that the mind absorbs knowledge and is influenced by thoughts dependent on the context where a person sees his. It is evident by the variety of personalities individuals show at various stages of their lives. Parents need to ensure that their children are raised in settings that foster positive mental development throughout their lives. Children who have the chance to have a positive upbringing when they were children are more likely to live decent lives. The brain and memory of an individual are always working on various tasks. It is essential to know the different states of the brain while analyzing information about how brain function.

The brain's right and left hemispheres have distinct hemispheres. Every component in the brain plays a role in how our body functions in a holistic way. Based on studies it is believed that the right brain's hemisphere regulates the left part of the body. On the other hand, the left hemisphere regulates the right-hand part of our body. Anyone who wants to make an ad-hoc joke on this issue could argue that our mental processes are designed to work in conjunction with the other. However, when they delve deeper into this joke could discover that the joke has a lot of logic.

The brain's neurons create a complex system which allows communications. The brain cells use small electric charges to transfer information from one nerve to the next. The term "nerve system" refers to the entire physiological system which contain neurons. Each function of the brain in the nervous system is responsible for bringing the state that is intangible for the brain, referred to as the mind to existence. The mind process thoughts, emotions, and emotions since they are the primary languages that which the brain comprehends.

The conscious state of mind is called the conscious state within the mind. The mind can be classified in two different states, aware and unconscious. According to research the conscious brain analyzes only 10% of the event, while the subconscious mind manages the remaining 90%. However the mind of each is dependent on each other and can't function independently of one. The subconscious mind lies under the conscious one and the limited access helps to guard against harmful thoughts.

The mind and memory work together in order to influence different brain activity. The memory that is not good for one particular action will always cause people to avoid the situation however a positive memory of the same activity makes one appreciate it, and to develop a frequent predisposition to the activity. It is essential to lead an ideal lifestyle in order to determine the standards that society consider favorable and negative criteria.

The brain of a human is one of the largest organs of the human body because it differentiates us from all other living species living on earth. Humans are more intelligent than others due to their capacity to process, think and comprehend information. Brains are the primary nervous system that runs throughout our body. It is inextricably connected to any physiological change that include stress. Stress, as per experts, can have an effect on memory as well as capacity to organize. In addition, studies are currently taking place to find out which part of the brain gets affected by stress, so that it is able to be managed.

Stress Processing in the Brain

Human bodies are complex and intricate in its chemical reactions. If someone is under stress it triggers numerous chemical reactions. While stress can be helpful in situations of physical danger, it triggers an emotional response within the body. In the end, having this level of stress often can cause harm. But in our stressed-out society, such a situation is not a choice.

What effects do stress on your brain and body? To live, a range of biological responses to stress in supplying oxygen and blood to the vital organs. This means that when trying to deal with the threat, different bodily functions are neglected. The brain releases chemicals that trigger changes due to the events that occur in a stressful circumstance. The chemicals that are that are released into bloodstreams include adrenalin, cortisol, noradrenaline, as well as endorphins.

How Does Stress Affect Brain Function?

In light of the fact that stress has been proven to impact brain function it is important to consider which components of brain function change in response to stress events. The degree of effect the stress type has on the brain is contingent upon how immediate it is or over a period of time. In the case of stress, however, memory is the area of the brain that is affected most.

The effects of stress have been demonstrated to cause damage to short-term memory in the spoken word. If you're constantly under stress, the capacity you have to recall information has been significantly decreased, and you might be unable to focus on your job or remember important information. The loss of memory is significantly more for older people who are stress-prone. The loss of memory in these conditions is, as per research findings it was due to the loss of the hippocampus consequence of elevated cortisol levels. The same gland that controls the memory of your body.

Stress Management

There's an array of methods that can assist you with stress regardless of how intense the situation. Regular exercises and meditation are proven to alleviate stress through the release of muscle tension. Additionally, other practical measures to reduce stress like better time managing and organizational skills can be very helpful, whether in the workplace or at home.

MYTHS ABOUT THE BRAIN

The brain is among the most vital and fascinating organs found in our body. It is responsible for the nervous system of our central nerves. It assists us in breathing, thinking talk, move, and speak. The brain, which is home to approximately 100 billion neurons is a very complex organ. Due to the complexity of the brain it is a subject to many fields of science and medicine have been devoted to research and treatment of the brain, such as neurology, that treats brain-related physical disorders and psychology, which focuses on how people behave and their mental processes as well as psychological medicine that addresses mental illnesses. These two fields, along with specific components from each are more likely to overlap with deeper research into the brain.

The brain's structure isn't entirely understood, proving the truth about it is a particular challenge. But, over the last few decades, a variety of researchers have conducted enough research to debunk a number of common beliefs about the brain. Scientists have discovered facts about the psychological aspects of the brain behaviour, behaviors, and interrelations with motivational variables, as well as specific details. Researchers also discovered debunkings of commonly held brain-related theories.

A myriad of misconceptions surround the brain. However, only a handful of facts are based on fact. A few of the authors debunk commonly held beliefs about the brain, and provide extensive, valuable knowledge about how the brain functions.

Combining cutting-edge research with spiritual teachings, removing the most common brain-related myths which limit our abilities while laying out how to:

Develop the best lifestyle you can for your body and mind.

Enhance happiness and wellbeing by encouraging physical and mental well-being as well as addressing the pressing concerns, like anxiety, mental health obesity, depression and reducing the dangers of ageing.

Instead of letting your mind to dictate your actions, make use of the power of your brain instead.

The brain is capable of remarkable healing and rebuilding. The brain that is alive, throbbing which is located in our bones on the other hand, is covered in white or black. It is also red, in addition to being an unappealing, dull shade of gray. The brain's myth is not unique to other stories, but has some truth.

It is good to know that a new generation researchers and physicians is able to dispel commonly held beliefs about the brain, and giving us incredibly valuable knowledge about how the brain operates. Another among the most popular misconceptions concerning the brain and ageing is that, as we grow more mature, our brains alter and are less healthful. The vast amount of research regarding the psychological effects of aging suggests that specific cognitive processes are drastically altered when people get older.

Chapter 3: How To Keep Your Mind Sharp Throughout Your Life

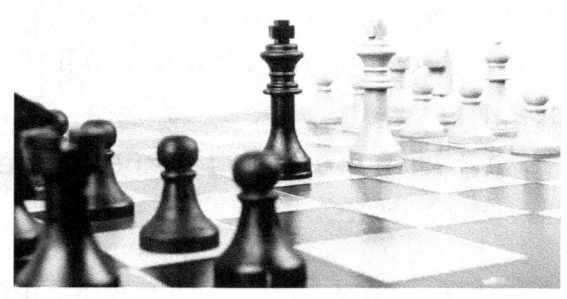

Everyone experiences an (senior time) at least once in a while. There are times when you enter the kitchen with no idea the reason, or abandon your keys. Though these mental issues are annoying, they don't require a trip at the physician. The most frequent physical problems are blood pressure issues or discomfort and incapacitation however if your mental well-being isn't in good shape then your physical health may be affected as well.

Research suggests that pursuing certain health habits that seem to be simple could increase the capacity of your brain's memory and reduce the risk of getting mad. Are you already past your prime? Be assured. As per research it is true that brains continue to create new connections with age. The eight strategies listed below will assist you in achieving that.

Learn to speak a different language The process of learning a second (or the third) language, as per the findings of a recent study, can expose the brain to unusual cognitive challenges and could delay your development in dementia. Let's say you find that the Spanish name for mom is "Madre." It may be difficult initially to remember that phrase, but after a few repetitions the word will begin to be embedded within your lexicon. This simple memory indicates that your brain has created an entirely new pathway. Each week, you should set aside the evening for you to either speak (however unspoken) in a language you have never heard of or just to be silent and use the sign language.

Engage in a sport you have never tried before The mental stress of activities helps to build up a brainpower reserve that can be used over the course of years. Naturally, finding a new passion that you are interested in is vital. You can take up gardening, play you can learn how to play an instrument. If you do decide to take up any of these, make sure it's an exciting experience for you. If you're skilled in word searches, you can try them as an alternative to a crossword. Are you interested in writing tasks? You might want to try sketching or painting.

Foods that boost brain function A diet that is rich in vegetables, fruits, and whole grain foods, as well as that are low in saturated fat may assist in helping to keep brain cells healthy. A variety of healthy food items, including nuts, fruits, and vegetables or fatty fish, of course, a daily glass of wine is proven in research studies to increase your cognitive capacity as well as encourage the development of new brain cells and stop mental decline. Put a handful of snacks in your purse or in your glove compartment. Your brain requires regular nourishment to ensure optimal performance (at minimum every three to 5 hours).

Exercise: Exercising has been repeatedly proven to improve the functioning of the brain, especially on areas that are involved in the process of learning as well as memory. But don't worry. It doesn't take more than an hour in the gym to experience the advantages of exercise for improving your cognitive function. Participating in any activity (such such as cycling, running or walking) for a period of

30 minutes each day will help to increase your blood flow into the brain. Based on preliminary research results, the benefits from physical activity are most apparent when it's you add a mental exercise. This means that activities such as taking part in a dancing class, learning about a new martial art and practicing yoga can be particularly useful.

Sleep in and catch sleep: getting enough sleep is among the most beneficial things you can do to improve your brain. Although sleep is essential for your mind and body to function, experts do not know what takes place during the time you sleep. The benefits of sleep are improved memory and better learning through the renewal of cell walls and eliminating excess brain waste. It is important to try and get 7-8 hours of sleep each evening. Are you struggling to get 8 hours of restful sleep? Through the day, you can take energy naps.

Keep an eye on your medical conditions: Keeping healthful body and mind can help protect your brain as well as your body. There are a variety of medical ailments like diabetes, depression as well as high blood pressure and hypothyroidism can affect the brain's capacity to function. Your memory can be protected by following the doctor's prescriptions, following your doctor's orders exactly as prescribed, and logging any change in the brain's function.

Do some sort of meditation The need for a break is crucial to allow the brain to recuperate and reflect. In fact, research has shown the fact that "thinking about not being thinking" is beneficial in both mental and physical wellbeing. In addition, research indicates that regular meditation can enhance memory. For 10 or 15 minutes a morning to clear your mind, and solely focusing upon your breathing. It will not just let your mind rest and relax, but your focused breathing can also boost the blood flow to it.

In order to maintain relationships with your loved ones, it requires some mental ability. It's not just about communication that requires rapid thinking, but also is settling disputes, and analyzing current events. According to studies Socially-engaged elders might be more likely to develop Alzheimer's disease than wallflower peers. Build relationships with other people across all age groups, races and ethnicities in order to enhance your mental workload you can do. When trying to understand the differences in tone, speech or even some of the latest cultural terms your brain could be challenged to create new connections.

Chapter 4: Brain-Healthy Foods To Increase Brain Power

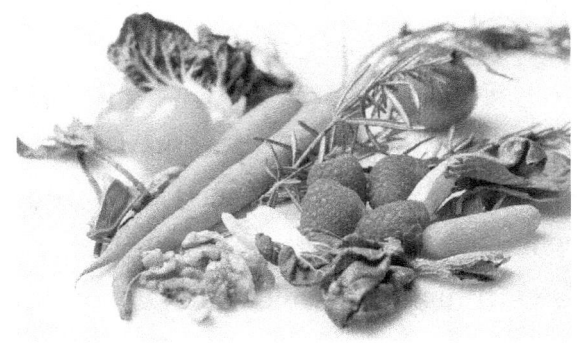

Different meals could provide the necessary nutrients for enhancing brain power. Here are some foods that can help improve cognitive functioning. An eating plan rich with omega fatty acids as an example, can boost the activity of nerve cells, and help keep blood vessels within the brain uncongested. Fish consumption, which is abundant in omega-3 fatty acids every week at least two times can help with this.

It is essential to be aware of the kinds of foods that could boost brain functioning and those foods that can affect brain performance. Opioids and alcohol, as an example, can severely harm the brain cells. Additionally, certain foods may block an artery, which could result in a decrease in circulation of blood towards the brain. Foods with high glycemic index can create dangerous fluctuations in blood sugar which can cause anxiety in the body and brain.

The vitamins and minerals on this list must be consumed daily for your brain to work properly.

The fruits include cantaloupe, bananas as well as oranges and avocados.

The most popular vegetables include the collard greens, broccoli, potato, spinach, peas, romaine lettuce and.

Whole grain products comprise oats, wheat, and brown rice.

Dairy foods include cheese eggs, milk as well as yogurt.

The protein-rich foods comprise chicken, turkey as well as salmon and tuna.

Contrarily those foods that cause harm for brain health include alcohol sugar, corn syrup, the frosting industry, synthetic sweeteners artificial food colorings sugar, sweets from junk food white bread smoking, hydrogenated oils and eating too much.

In the past, it was stated that alcohol can cause brain damage in a flash and nicotine may cause capillaries that constrict, restricting circulation to the brain. The consumption of hydrogenated fats has been connected to the development of cardiovascular disease and obstruction of the arterial system. In order to improve brain functioning take every step to limit, or even completely avoid the intake of brain-damaging foods.

It is therefore essential to take advantage of more the brain-healthy foods, which are complex carbs which provide an unstoppable fuel source. Be aware that the way you cook and consume food affects your body and brain. The protein-rich food you eat can improve brain activity by providing amino acids needed to make neurotransmitters. Neurotransmitters act as messengers between brain cells. The higher the quality of these messengers to the brain, the greater efficiency the brain performs.

Chapter 5: Aphasia (A Neurological Condition)

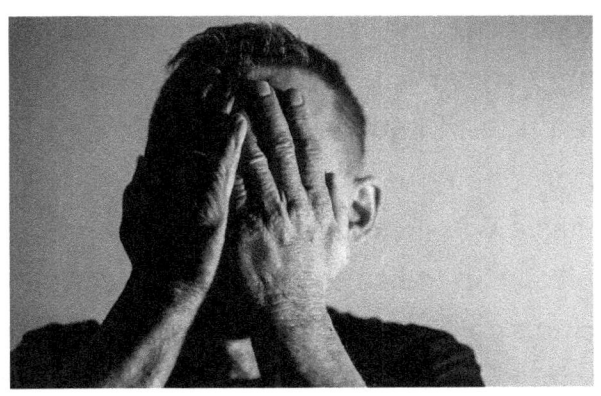

Aphasics sufferers have difficulties communicating or hearing people talk. As a result of a neurological issue this happens because the brain areas that govern spoken language get injured or damaged. This is usually the case with other disorders, like stroke. As aphasia tends to be curable however, therapy for speech may aid those suffering from it for the rest of their lives.

This usually occurs because a portion of your brain has been damaged, however it can be triggered by circumstances that affect how the brain functions. Aphasia manifests in a variety of different ways. The place of injury within your brain is the determining factor for what kind of aphasia you'll experience. The condition is typically an indication of another condition including stroke or brain injury. Sometimes, it can be an occasional side effect from ailments like migraines. It is usually treatable especially when the condition can be treated or is a good outcome.

What is the difference between dysphasia and dysarthria as well as the apraxia?

Other disorders of speech and that have a connection and/or overlap to aphasia are dysphasia, dysarthria, as well as Apraxia.

Aphasia is a broad term that refers to a brain-related issue that affects language skills that include difficulty communicating or understanding others. The term is used by experts to describe a complete or a partial loss in linguistic capabilities. Dysphasia was a term from the past which refers to the loss of language capabilities that is caused by a brain-related disorder. The term "dysphasia" isn't often employed in all locations. Its possibility of being misinterpreted as "dysphagia" is the main reason for its declination of use. Dysphagia is a medical term used to describe difficulty in swallowing. The muscles involved in swallowing are required to force food, liquids as well as other substances into your throat. Dysphagia can be due to problems in the brain, nervous system, or the muscles themselves.

Dysarthria occurs when you experience difficulties speaking because of problems with the respiratory system of your upper your mouth, or even your face. In the result, you might speak with irregular rates, or with blurred or disorganized pronunciations, or that you have unusually high or low pitch (changing between highand high-pitched voice). Apraxia can cause difficulties with tasks that you've done before or in which you've acquired the necessary skills. As an example, you might discover that you are unable to utilize a key for opening the door even though you know how to do it and you are well-versed in how locks and keys function. People with apraxia may are unable to pronounce words correctly.

Aphasia can be a problem for anyone with brain damage. the regions of the brain which control the ability of a person to communicate or hear the words of others. Though it could be experienced at any age but it's most common for people who are middle aged and older particularly as a result of stroke-related diseases.

What's the incidence of this condition?

The condition is rare which affects two millions people across a few regions of the world. There are more than 180,000 patients diagnosed every year. This is a frequent occurrence under specific situations. A prime example of this is stroke, in which aphasia is a problem that affects nearly one third of people who suffer from the disorder.

What are the effects of this disease to my body?

The people with this disorder often feel that people are difficult to comprehend them due to it affects their ability to talk. This can lead to a variety of difficulties. Small inconveniences, like not being able to ask for the water you need or request a drink of water, are examples. Some other mistakes, for instance the inability to inform others your stroke-related symptoms, can be life-threatening.

What are the signs and symptoms that are associated with the condition of aphasia?

Aphasia and other related disorders may have a wide range of manifestations. There are many commonalities with aphasia-related symptoms however, there are some important distinctions. In order to understand the way aphasia functions must be first understood two distinct brain regions that are involved to speak:

The Broca's region was named for Broca's area was named after the French physician who realized that this area of the brain is responsible for controlling the muscles that enable the person to speak. It's an area of the frontal lobe which's located on your left side right in front of the temple. The Wernicke's Territories: This part of the brain has been named in honor of Wernicke, a German neurologist who realized the brain's ability to regulate your ability to recognize and select words to speak. It's a region of the temporal lobe, which can be found mostly on the left side of your body located just above the ears.

Both parts of the brain collaborate in order to let you talk. Before transferring signals to the Broca's region Wernicke's area analyzes the language you comprehend and chooses the words to choose. Once Broca's area has decided what words to be used, signals are delivered to your muscles that which you speak with.

The Primary Types of Aphasia

The experts consider three main factors to determine the kind of aphasia someone has. There are eight types of aphasia. The elements that make up these are:

Fluency: Do they possess an easy, smooth sound? Does the tone, tempo as well as the pronunciation and grammar used in their speeches appropriate? Are they able to write with ease? Understanding. Does one comprehend what other people are speaking? If they speak, do they make use of coherent sentences and words? They are able to read and comprehend the written words. Repetition. Does the person having difficulty repetition of words, phrases or even sentences?

The aphasia of Broca

The most frequent kinds of this disease is (expressive Aphasia) sometimes referred to "non-fluent theosis." The condition is often seen in people with the following symptoms:

Drop in fluency Patients suffering from Broca's Aphasia are unable to form the words. As they struggle or become not able to recall the words you speak to them, they might repeat the same words or sentences in short phrases again. Mutism, which is the ability to create only one sound at one time can occur in the most extreme varieties. It is not a problem for comprehension. People with Broca's aphasia may be not able to speak, however they are able to hear what other people say. Additionally, they are able to identify the signs of speech problems. The difficulty of repetition is. Since it affects the repetition process, people who suffers from Broca's Aphasia might be unable to repeat the words you say to them.

Other indicators The damage to the Broca's region most commonly from strokes frequently affects the neighboring area of the brain which controls muscle action. In turn, those who suffer from Broca's aphasia may be more likely to suffer from weakness on the opposite side of their bodies.

Aphasia-like Wernicke

Aphasia of this kind is quite common and is known in the form of (fluent Aphasia) or "receptive anaphasia." Wernicke's Aphasia can affect people with the following characteristics:

Talking clearly: This indicates that they do not have physical problem speaking. However, they do frequently speak in a manner that is unnatural or inexplicably bizarre. People who have it might create new terms or employ inappropriate words. Some experts call this the "word salad." It is difficult to comprehend. Individuals with this type of condition struggle to understand what people can say. They may be able to understand simple sentences. However, the more complex the word or phrase is that to grasp. The ability to repeat words is an issue. Since it hinders repetition, people with Wernicke's Aphasia could have trouble attempting to repeat speech or phrases given to them. Additional indications. The Wernicke's brain is situated near to regions of the brain which affect vision. Hence, people suffering from the condition often have vision issues. Aphasic patients with Wernicke's syndrome often suffer from anosognosia. This is a condition where the brain is unable to discern or recognize signs of an issue with your health. This is why people who suffer from this type of aphasia may be unaware of it or do not realize that they are suffering from it.

Complete aphasia

It is the most serious type of the condition known as aphasia. It is common for these components to be found.

Drop in fluency: People with global aphasia may find it hard to communicate with a high volume of. Most severe cases could cause a person to create extremely weak or isolated noises, or not make any sound even (mutism). The person may also repeat simple words or phrases. They will be less fluent as they are unable to understand what you are saying to them. trouble understanding. The people who suffer from this issue are unable to comprehend what other people have to say. They may be able to understand simple sentences. However, the more complicated the phrase or language becomes, the harder it becomes to comprehend. The difficulty of repetition is. Someone who suffers from global aphasia might be unable to recall the words or phrases they say to you. Other indicators: This type of aphasia can result from conditions which can cause significant brain injury including severe head injuries or strokes. The damage usually affects many parts of the brain. It can be severe, leading to blindness, one-sided paralysis along with other serious issues.

Alternative types of Aphasia

Transcortical Motor Aphasia is comparable to Broca's Aphasia. However, it is it is less severe. A notable distinction is that those affected by this condition have no difficulty with repeating phrases or words that are spoken to them. The Wernicke's Aphasia may be similar to transcortical sensory aphasia however, it's not as severe. People who suffer from it, as do those suffering from transcortical motor aphasia are not able to repeat the words you speak. Aphasia of this kind occurs in brain degenerative conditions like Alzheimer's disease. Aphasia of the conductor affects fluency, but does not impact comprehension. Patients with this condition struggle to pronounce words, particularly when being you ask them to repeat what they have said. People with mixed transcortical aphasia in contrast to those who suffer from global aphasia may be able to repeat the words of others around them. Anomic aphasia: Those with such aphasia experience difficulties in coming up with phrases specifically words used to define objects or activities.

It is common for them to use several words for communicating their message. They may also use broad language such as "object" to overcome the issue. There are other conditions similar to or comprise the condition of aphasia. Aphasia Progressive Primary (PPA). Although it is not a word it is not a disease, it's a condition which affects the brain's degenerative. The people suffering from the condition slowly lose their capacity to speak in a vocal manner, whether it be through writing, reading as well as orally. It is different from aphasia that occurs through a stroke or accident that does not get worse over time. PPA can manifest different manners, such as frontotemporal dementia as well as Alzheimer's disease.

Agraphia and the condition of word vision (alexia) (inability to type). Abrasions to parts of your brain which affect speech could affect your ability to write and read. While people who have alexia are able to detect words, they are unable to comprehend or read these words. Agraphia sufferers aren't able to write. Though both disorders can be co-existent, it's extremely rare to find someone with alexia and not have agraphia. This is why they are able to write however they are unable to read what they've created. Auditory verbal agnosia is the condition where one can listen to other talking but can't distinguish the sound from their own voice. This happens because the brain's processing of sounds or spoken words gets disrupted.

Aphasia can be caused by any illness that affects the brain. The condition could also be due to issues in the brain's functions. Here are a few possibilities for the cause:

Alzheimer's disease.

Aneurysms.

Activity in the brain.

The brain is a target for cancer (including brain cancer).

Hypoxia in the brain (brain destruction due to a the lack of oxygen).

Concussion and trauma can cause damage to the brain.

Frontotemporal and dementia with dementia.

Congenital disorders as well as developmental disorders (diseases which occur during birth due to an error in the fetal development).

Seizures or epilepsy (especially the case where they result in permanent brain injury).

Genetic disorders are diseases that are present at birth and are passed down from either one or both of your parents. For example, Wilson's disease.

The brain is inflamed (encephalitis) is the result of virus, bacteria, or autoimmune conditions.

Migraines (this affect is temporary) (this affect is not permanent).

Chemotherapy and radiation therapy are two options.

Poisons and toxins (such in carbon monoxide poisoning, or the poisoning of heavy metals).

Strokes or transient assaults (TIAs).

Are they contagious?

Aphasia is not a common occurrence. Though many diseases can trigger it however none of them can cause aphasia. To determine if you have aphasia, an examination of your body, questions regarding your medical history, diagnostic tests and imaging, as well as various other methods are utilized. If necessary an expert in medicine could recommend a set of tests in order to identify other conditions or triggers of symptoms that are similar to the ones caused by Aphasia. Below are some examples:

Tests for sensory and neurologic function. Tests will show the fact that an aphasia-like condition does not result from issues with hearing or nerve damage.

Memory and Cognitive Assessments. These tests will ensure that a test results indicate that the person's cognitive capabilities or memory do not pose a problem.

Diagnostic and imaging processes. They look for abnormalities or indications of brain injury within the region affected.

If doctors suspect aphasia they might conduct a series of tests. A speech pathologist is able to aid in determining what type of aphasia the person has or has. The results of tests could also be used to identify the root cause for the disorder and the most effective method for treatment.

Test options can include:

A blood test (these could reveal anything including immune system issues to poisons and toxins, specifically certain metals, such as copper).

An CT scan is a type that uses computed tomography.

EEG stands for electroencephalogram (EEG).

Electromyogram.

The possibility was assessed.

Magnetic resonance imaging (MRI) for the analysis of genetics (MRI).

PET scan is also referred to as positron emission.

Retapping (lumbar puncture).

X-rays.

Can aphasia be treated and how can it be treated?

There is currently no treatment for Aphasia. But, it's usually addressed in some manner. The first step to treat aphasia usually is to deal with the root cause. The speedy restoration of blood flow into the affected part of the brain can help to prevent or reduce long-term injury in diseases like stroke.

It is common for aphasia to be temporary if it is caused by a short-term issue, such as concussion, migraine, seizures or ailment. In the majority of cases, once you heal and your brain heals result of your treatments and time your aphasia gets better or is completely eliminated.

If an individual has sustained serious brain injury that's lasting or long-lasting treatment, speech therapy could assist them to regain their linguistic capabilities. The therapies can also assist the patient develop better social skills as well as compensatory strategies to overcome their speech aphasia. Families and friends could also participate in speech therapy to talk to you and support you in the best way they can.

The drugs or treatment options employed to treat conditions which cause aphasia can vary in a significant way. Therefore the healthcare provider can be the most reliable source for knowledge about the different treatments which can help you. Therapies can be adapted to meet your particular requirements and situation. The medical issues or personal preferences that could affect the course of treatment will be taken into consideration. It is possible to experience problems or side effects based on the cause of your illness at the beginning as well as the treatment you are using. The doctor who treats you may explain the many side effects and problems that may occur to be encountered in your particular circumstance. It is also important to inquire regarding what you could take to prevent or mitigate adverse effects.

Aphasia may be an indicator of serious brain damage or impairment. Aphasia-related diseases are very serious and some can be dangerous to your life. In the end that you shouldn't attempt to diagnose yourself with aphasia. If you or someone else you have with you is experiencing symptoms akin to aphasia dial your emergency phone number as soon as possible so you are able to receive medical care.

Aphasia recovery times vary depending on the cause of the illness, the length of time it will last and the treatment used. Your doctor will be the most qualified person to provide the details about how long it'll be to get better and heal.

Patients with aphasia have a variety of options in taking better care of themselves and dealing with the effects of it.

People with aphasia can be able to take care of themselves through the following actions:

Talk to your physician according to the instructions.

Regular check-ups can help you monitor your health, and work to lessen the effects of your illness.

Following the treatment guidelines of your physician.

Following the prescribed dosage as well as visiting a speech therapist are two ways to go (if your doctor would recommend the therapy).

Try to join support groups as often as possible. The support groups you join, whether in person or on the internet could help you to learn about other patients with aphasia. Patients with aphasia are often isolated or lonely because their ability to communicate affected.

Discover other ways of communicating. The writing process allows those with Aphasia to communicate since it involves parts of the brain that tend to be untapped, especially for those suffering from Broca's aphasia.

Technology can be beneficial. Mobile devices, like tablets and smartphones can help people who have aphasia by giving them more verbal and nonverbal ways of communicating. They also come with apps specifically designed for those with aphasia.

Make sure you carry a label that states you are aphasic. Aphasia identification or a card will allow you to communicate with those who aren't sure the identity of you or whether they have an aphasia.

What could I do to aid my loved ones who suffer from Aphasia?

Many options are readily available to people who have loved ones who has the condition known as aphasia. Certain of these suggestions can aid your loved one to connect and improve their communication while aiding in their daily life. They can also help with recovering or managing their illness. The tasks you could perform include:

Take your time and be patient Give your loved one with aphasia to have a space and time to talk. Help them feel secure and energized. Give them the freedom to complete their sentences without stopping while letting them fail without correction. If they want help, offer it to them but allow them to try it independently initially.

Seek out opportunities for interaction. Aphasia interferes with communication, and often leads to intense feelings of isolation and loneliness. It is possible to have a positive influence when you talk to your beloved in a manner that's easy and relaxing for the person.

It is easier for people to talk between themselves: Grab their attention before beginning talking, keep eye contact, pay all your attention to them as well as, if any time possible, cut down on the background sound (such as turning off your television). If they are interested and find it beneficial, provide them with other ways of communicating, like drawing, writing hand gestures, writing and using devices that are smart. Respect and treat them with respect. Patients with an aphasia can be ashamed or embarrassed by their difficulties with communication.

Help them to be treated your children with respect and dignity In the event that your children are not understanding your words and your words, you can try introducing them to shorter ones or phrases. Also If they are more comfortable, inquire about their preferences. Do not speak to your children in a disrespectful or loud tone or talking in a slow manner. Additionally, unless specifically directed to do so, refrain not speaking more loudly. What is the best time to seek medical treatment?

If you're beginning to notice symptoms of aphasia you must take care of your medical needs as soon as is possible. If you notice that your symptoms are getting worse it is recommended that you consult the doctor. It could be a sign of a brain disease that is degenerative instead of injuries or damages caused due to a medical condition, such as stroke.

Chapter 6: Brain Fog

The symptoms of brain fog include the inability to focus, confusion, and an absence of focus as well as mental clarity. The stress of work, the lack of sleep as well as stress and the use of excessive technology could be the cause. The brain fog can be the result of excessive levels of inflammation within the cell and also changes in the hormones responsible for controlling your energy level, mood as well as your attention. Insufficient levels of hormones in a state of imbalance affect the entire system. In the wake of this syndrome, different issues such as the irregularity of menstrual flow, obesity and diabetes mellitus could arise.

The medical issue isn't commonly referred to as "brain fog." It is a set of signs that can hinder the ability to think. It is possible to feel lost or overwhelmed, have difficulty to concentrate, or experience difficulties putting your thoughts into the right words. A lot of pregnant women complain about being unable to remember details. While pregnant, lots of physical changes take place and the substances that are secreted to safeguard and nourish the unborn baby can exacerbate memory issues.

Since it impacts your central nervous system it can affect how the mind "talks" towards the other parts of your body. Most MS sufferers have issues related to attention, memory to detail, language, or planning. Memory and learning exercises can help therapy, as well as therapists can provide you with new strategies for your issues.

A few prescription and non-prescription drugs can affect your mental clarity. If you're on medication and find that you're being as clear as you would like to or you've lost your mental clarity, talk to your physician. Be sure to inform them about every drug you are taking. The medical community is divided about whether the sensitivity of certain chemicals (both made and natural) can cause brain fog.

Chemotherapy is a powerful drugs-based treatment for cancer, could be the cause of "chemo brain" in the sense it's commonly referred to. It is possible that you have trouble managing multiple tasks, recalling details such as dates, names or finding it difficult to finish the tasks. While it is usually gone quickly, a few sufferers may experience symptoms over a prolonged time after treatment. In the case of cancer, for instance, if it has affected the brain area this could caused "brain fog."

As women get older it is possible that they have trouble recalling new information or finding it difficult to learn. This happens around the age of 50, which is about one year following their last menstrual cycle.

The hot flashes, that are frequent occurrences of sweating, and a subsequent increase in body temperature and heart rate, are also possible. Certain forms of treatment like hormone supplements, could be beneficial. When you suffer from this illness your mind and body are likely to feel tired over a long time. You may feel overwhelmed, forgetful and irritable. Although there's no proven cure for CFS medication, medications or talk therapy can assist.

It is possible that you don't be able to recall information well or the ability to deal with problems quickly. It's not easy to know the cause of this, whether it's lack of motivation or energy caused by melancholy, or whether depression causes an impact on your brain that creates a fog. By taking medication as well as talk therapy to treat your depression, you'll be able to return in the right direction.

The need for sleep is necessary for the brain to function effectively, however excessive sleep can cause you to become drowsy. Try to get 7 to nine hours. Do not drink or consume alcohol following dinner or before going to sleeping, and having your laptop and smartphone in your bedroom could aid you to sleep more comfortably. Sleeping in and getting up around the identical time each day could prove beneficial. Talk to your doctor in case you suspect that an sleep issue, such as sleep apnea, insomnia or narcolepsy is creating the brain to fog up.

It's normal to feel nervous and confused in certain instances, particularly during situations of intense tension. The people who claim anxiety and confusion are affecting in their daily activities, however it is recommended to see a physician.

What is the cause of stress and how does it affect thinking?

Anxiety Saps Mental Vitality.

It might take greater energy to concentrate not on something other than anxious thoughts. People may think that anxiety can affect the ability to think clearly. In the end, they could be harder to focus and concentrate. The effects of anxiety can vary on an individual's performance based upon the work being performed and in relation to the level of brain fog.

The researchers exposed their participants to a set of tension-inducing tasks. Researchers found that anxiety made it more difficult for tasks, which made these tasks harder. The effects of anxiety on the more challenging actions were less noticeable.

Researchers suggest it is due to the tough task required more brain resources and left less room to worry. The researchers aren't sure whether a similar situation could happen in stress-related scenarios that are actually occurring.

The stress of anxiety can affect your ability to think clearly and cause confusion in the brain. What needs to be completed can make people feel more nervous. A person who's taking care of their home or filing taxes for instance could discover new causes to worry. It could increase anxiety as well as cause cognitive fog and make more difficult to accomplish their task.

Brain fog and anxiety can result from the following problems with mental health:

Depression as well as attention deficit hyperactivity disorders as well as anxiety disorders like generalized anxiety disorder (GAD) and Post-traumatic anxiety disorder (PTSD) are just a few types of mental disorders (ADHD)

Health issues can create anxiety or cognitive fog.

Symptoms of Brain fog

The symptom of brain fog is and not a diagnosis. Individuals may have varying experiences and utilize the same word to describe a variety of signs. Here are some signs of brain fog

Neurological diseases like dementia and Alzheimer's along with head injuries, can be due to food scarcity and dehydration or vitamin deficiency.

Lupus is a chronic disease that can be treated with and alcohol, as well as illegal substances such as lupus and a variety of medications such as chemotherapy, are just a few instances of drugs.

Brain Stroke

A stroke, often referred to as a stroke, happens the moment a blood vessel inside the brain breaks or ruptures, or something blocks blood flow into a specific region within the brain. The reason for this could be the following two factors: the artery is blocked or breaking.

In any case, the parts of the brain have been injured or have degenerated. Patients suffering from strokes may experience lifelong disabilities, brain damage or even die.

What's the effect of a brain injury? brain?

Our emotions, thoughts as well as our speech all originate from the brain. It is also responsible for our daily activities and also stores memories. The brain is also responsible for many different physical systems like digestion and breathing.

To operate properly, your brain needs oxygen. The blood vessels provide oxygen-rich blood supply to each area of the brain. As they're starved of oxygen, the brain cells start to die in a matter of minutes following the obstruction of blood flow. This is why the risk of a stroke increases. The serious medical condition demands immediate intervention.

The different types of Strokes For example.

They are divided into two categories:

Ischemia-related stroke.

Stroke hemorrhagic.

An ischemic transient attack is typically referred to"mini-stroke" or "mini-stroke" (TIA). Brain blood flow is shut off for a much shorter time that in other forms of stroke, typically less than 5 minutes.

The cause of schizophrenia-related stroke is schizophrenia.

Chapter 7: Diet

As soon as your brain begins becoming "fuzzy" you may be thinking, "Did I eat something unusual?" The answer could to be "yes," so you might be correct in asking the inquiry. When I refer to "diet," I'm not talking about Atkins, Keto, Paleo and Raw Vegan. I'm using the word "diet" simply as a broad term to describe the foods you consume inside your body. It is not necessary to to adhere to a particular trendy eating plan. Any diet that isn't sustainable for you regardless of whether it is to be beneficial, won't do much good over the long haul. In deciding on your personal "diet," it's good generally to pick what you're able to sustain for a lifetime as well as it's totally acceptable to choose and decide the one that works for you but not feeling pressured to become a member of a specific eating plan.

It is very likely that what you're taking in isn't ideal for you mind. The most widely-known "culprits" that cause your mental anxiety could be due to sugar, fast-burning carbohydrates and caffeine MSG as well as foodstuffs. Problems with fast burning sugars, carbs as well as caffeine is that they're consumed by the body in a rapid manner which can result in either a physical or mental increase in energy that is that is then followed by a crash. Caffeine specifically, functions as a stimulant creating a vicious circle as the release of caffeine triggers withdrawal symptoms. It is possible that you have to cut these substances out completely based on how they impact you personally. The bodies of different people react differently to the identical items. Some people is enough to decrease some things. For others, it might be required to completely eliminate certain items completely.

If you're eating foods which you're allergic or intolerable to, it's another case in which you'll need to cut out certain foods from your menu. There are many people who suffer from unknown allergies over time without knowing they have it. It's simple to imagine things that trigger extreme or apparent reactions as being allergies (for example, your throat getting swollen after eating nuts, or breaking out in itchy hives after eating shellfish) But allergies could cause a subtle in-depth effect on our bodies. If you consume foods that your body is having a tough time making sense of, energy is diverted from the brain, instead focusing to digestion. While what you see on the outside could appear to an allergy of a small amount or a non-existent allergy but on the inside, it could cause havoc to your brain. Hence, having an allergy test that is accurate and getting rid of the problematic foods is beneficial for your health.

But there are times when it's not about cutting out things, but is more of a need to include items. A lack of fats or drinking water can result in cognitive issues and therefore, you might have to boost these into your diet to improve the functioning to your brain.

If you're not looking to make drastic changes in your diet in a single day, the ideal option is to set aside a few weeks to write down all the food that you consume and what you're feeling. Choose one item or food type each time that you want to avoid or to add into your food regimen over a period of 3 to 10 days, to see if it affects your diet. The process can take time therefore don't try to rush the process. The process of eliminating and adding many things simultaneously will mean it is difficult to pinpoint exactly what causes the issue. If you follow this procedure correctly, and in time you'll start observe patterns and connections with certain food items, as well as the physical and mental state of your body.

If you're looking to get experts instead of figuring everything out by yourself You can consult an naturopathic physician, as well as an allergist.

Nutrition

There is a possibility that you could cut out those "bad" foods out of your diet, as described in the above section however, you may still suffer from mental fog. It could be due to deficiencies in the nutrition that you consume or absorb. If you're feeling as if that you're eating a healthy eating plan that consists of a majority of vegetables fruit, veggies, lean proteins, as well as other nutrient-rich whole meals, it is possible that your body's not taking in the nutrients contained in the food you consume. It can be frustrating when you're a health conscious person because you believe you're doing the proper things and making the right decisions, but there is no change despite the fact that have a healthy diet all the time.

It is here that enzymes, probiotics and supplements can be beneficial. A few of the most commonly-cited problems that cause the fog of your brain include Vitamin B12, Vitamin D and Omega-3 Fatty acids. There is the option of taking the supplements on your own or look for a multi-vitamin supplement that has appropriate levels of nutrients for your body. It is suggested that you take a multivitamin. Harvard School of Public Health considers multivitamins an "insurance program" for your health, in the event of a deficit in your nutrition. There is a reliable endorsement to take a multivitamin daily for proper brain function.

Alongside the commonly used vitamins and supplements to help your body and mind it is also worth including the following components which can aid in the mental acuity of your mind. They include:

Arctic root

Citicoline

Gotu Kola

Magnesium

Vinpocetine

Sleep

Another cause for Brain fog is that you aren't receiving sufficient sleep or getting enough sleep. If people are thinking of inadequate sleep most likely, they imagine insomnia or sleep Apnea. But there are over 70 sleep issues that can cause brain fog. Any one of they can result in the fog of your brain. Sleep is essential for health, and specifically, to your mental health. If you're sleeping your brain is basically cleansing itself, getting ready to start fresh the following day. If you aren't getting sufficient sleep the brain will not have the time to "sweep off the sand" or, as they say and prepare you to be clear the following day. Furthermore, sleep is the time when you save memories and develop new brain cells.

You can now see the reason sleep is essential. One night of low quality sleep could affect your memory, adversely affect your focus the following day, trigger emotional swings, impair your ability to judge, and reduce your ability to handle anxiety. Medical professionals and physicians even take the extreme step of compare a night of bad sleep to being legally impaired. This is the kind of effect sleep (or an absence of) could impact your thinking.

Stress

Contrary to what many believe the truth is that stress can be beneficial for your health. When you're being caught by a bear your body gets stressed out and can help you sharpen your concentration on getting out of the bear's path and staying alive. Being able to survive is good. Of course stress can be detrimental to your health, especially when it's in large levels or as a result of situations that are not life-threatening and are handled with a manner which does not really reflect the seriousness of what's occurring.

One example could be all the time stressed over your job. The body doesn't know what the distinction is between stress over work or due to running from a bear. Therefore, both situations will feel similar to you both emotionally and physically even though one is more important in comparison to the one. However, Western society doesn't help. The overwork that comes with it and the anxiety that comes with it are viewed as the result of a job done and a proof of productivity and hard work and a requirement for success.

However, continuously stressed is a risk of developing medical conditions that are serious at some point in the future. This includes the brain disorder dementia and Alzheimer's. Stress can also cause anxiety, depression, sleep issues, loss in memory, and diminished judgement, to mention just several. The longer you are suffering from constant stress, the more harm you can do to the brain.

One of the most effective techniques to lessen stress your life is to practice the practice of meditation. It's a good thing it's the right spot! The benefits of meditation are significant to your body and mind as well as reducing anxiety levels as well as clearing the brain's fog. You're not the only one. Meditation has been becoming increasingly more well-known within Western cultures and more than 20 million people living in the United States alone meditating on an ongoing basis.

There are many reasons to meditate. The US Marines have also instituted a meditation program to their troops, so If it's effective enough to assist the Marines manage anxiety, it could help people like you, and all the stresses that come with it. The other notable businesses that support the practice of meditation in their employees and employees comprise Proctor & Gamble, HBO, Nike, Apple, Google, Target, and General Mills. The practice has been proven to be an effective tool to help people deal with the stress of working in high-stress environments.

The practice of meditation reduces stress through enhancing your brain's ability manage difficult situations and to consider how you can best manage the situation. Also, it affects your mood and makes you feel happier over the long-run. Long-term practitioners also experience the improvement in their sleep and creativity levels as well as concentration and focus. Research has shown that meditation could reduce the age of your body by a tenth of a century! We'll get more specific regarding meditation in our next chapter. But due to its close connection to stress It was logical to include it in this short article.

Chapter 8: Physical Activity

The brain's food source is glucose and oxygen. When you're physically engaged, your body pumps out more endorphins. This results in additional glucose and oxygen into the brain. The result is a content brain. Furthermore, exercising can reduce stress levels by burning cortisol, a stress hormone. Therefore, engaging in some form of moderate or intense exercise every day of the week is among the most vital activities you can perform not just to improve the health of your brain, as well as for overall health.

Remember that exercising isn't required to be a constant workout every time to help your brain. small moments of energy are good for the brain. A thermogenesis process that doesn't require exercise is yet another method to lose weight to get your blood pumping and to engage physically active without an extra trip to the exercise studio. Walking is an excellent instance of a gentle to moderate activity that could help your brain to clear off the fog. Take your stairs instead of taking the elevator, ride a bike instead of driving and go for long walks. Little decisions like this each day can provide your brain with the benefit of exercise for your mind.

Toxin Exposure

This is a shocking number. In the last 100 years, over 800,00 new chemicals were developed. And, even more troublingly, among those chemicals, only five percent of them have been tested for human safety. This leaves an enormous amount of cleaners, pollutants as well as other substances in the air, making us vulnerable to potentially harmful negative effects to our minds and bodies. Within our own workplaces, homes as well as public spaces where the air is saturated with contaminants like smoke air fresheners, cleaning agents, pollen, mold or pet dander dust. The entire mess is stale within the air in and out of your house. Continuously inhaling this mix could cause mental fog and physical fatigue which can cause you to feel tired constantly. time.

There is no way to be in control of every situation you're in, but you may decide to live in a town that's recognized for its high air quality. You can invest into an air purifier for your home, switch out your cleansers with products which are greener that contain less harmful components, get rid of artificial air fresheners in your house in favour of essential oils and natural scents rather, and demand that your company implement the same change.

Health Conditions

The issue of having a fogged brain isn't linked to the lifestyle you choose, which is easy to manage and alter. In some cases, it's caused by a health issue. Actually, there numerous health issues that could affect your mental health. If you've ruled out significant lifestyle factors as the factor then it's time to consult your physician to conduct tests and dig into your symptoms in order to determine the cause behind the anxiety. Since it's frequent a medical adverse effect, it's typically classified according to the specific conditions or how to treat the issue. We come up with terms such as "Chemo Brain,"" "Lupus Fog" and "Thyroid Fog."

Medication

As brain fog can be an effect that is a result of certain health ailments, it can also be often a result of taking medications to treat the ailments. As an example, the drugs that are utilized to assist with sleeping or lower cholesterol levels are typically associated with memory loss. Many over-the-counter medicines could affect your ability to think clearly or concentration. Tylenol PM, Pepcid AC and Benadryl are just a handful of examples of over-the prescription medications that could alter your mental health. For almost any health issue there are a variety of medicines and brand names that can be found with various formulations, but still work and safe, which means that nothing is completely lost.

If you suffer from a medical issue that requires medication for treatment or suspect the medication you're taking isn't functioning properly on your mind, consult your physician regarding the symptoms you're experiencing, and ask them to prescribe another medication for you. If, for instance, you'd prefer not to depend on any medication or at all, consult an holistic physician to determine the possibility of treating your illness with natural remedies.

Introduction to Guided Meditation and Mindfulness

In some meditation circles and mindfulness, the concept of mindfulness is described as focusing on the goal, staying at the moment and not thinking about your thoughts and simply paying attention to the thoughts. Other practices employ mindfulness is regarded as keeping the focus present in the moment. These definitions provide concrete explanations for the meditation practice, as well as being similar to each other in that the emphasis is upon the act of taking action "on goal."

Each of these definitions defines mindfulness by referring to intent and deliberateness. Compare that to our normal way of living daily life and activities. The majority of our activities, like contemplating our daily routines or actions, occur in a way that is subconscious. We act on "autopilot." The practice of mindfulness can counterbalance these routine thinking patterns, and allows you to develop new habits of mind that bring greater clarity to your thoughts.

If you are constantly using "autopilot," it is it's like you're sleeping through the day. There is no time for enjoying every day beauty or individuals around your. Every day there is the chance to get up and take in completely in every second. The world is surrounding you and feel participant in it. It is possible to develop awareness. The ability to be a person rather than a watcher. This not only makes an ideal environment for living a fuller life, but it also does wonders in the brain and general well-being.

The International Journal of Wellbeing documented an investigation in 2016 that examined the benefits from MBSP, Mindfulness Based Strengths practice. The research was carried out on two participants: one group that had practiced MBSP while the other did not. The MBSP group who practiced was shown to show a substantial increase in the strength of their character, satisfaction, and involvement. This means that their psychological wellbeing dramatically enhanced.

The benefits from MBSP go beyond your personal life and into the workplace. If MBSP was implemented within a corporate setting to evaluate its effects on the organization, findings showed that after the managers and employees implemented MBSP and MBSP, they had the ability to solve issues and collaborate.

One of the easiest ways to become mindful throughout your day are engaging in activities such as paying all-in attention to the scent of the air on walking, the sensation of sand or grass under your feet, or even the sounds of the child's voice. Actually it's not only restricted to adults. If people can get started on the path towards mindfulness the more beneficial. The practice of encouraging children to be more conscious ultimately makes them adept at teaching, boosts their mental process and helps children to develop a confident view of themselves as they begin to concentrate more on their strengths and less so their weak points. There's also additional benefit from being aware of the present, which creates more memorable and memorable memories for the child as well as anyone else involved.

As you can see, regardless of age, mindfulness will positively affect the brain.

Its effects go far beyond the reduction of brain fog.

It's not a surprise, due to the nature being tied to the concept of consciousness and mindfulness, however being mindful increases your consciousness of the things that need to take place in your own life, as well as in the lives of people who are around you. It could be a great stimulus for self-improvement as well as development. As you will realize, applying awareness to your daily routine is worth the effort, at the very least.

Chapter 9: Guided Meditation

There are many different forms of meditation and forms, including "guided meditation" as one. It can be less daunting for people who are brand new to meditation. It is even more accessible to people who aren't experienced in meditation as there is someone who guides your meditation, offering guidance as well as making use of their voice to break up what could otherwise be silence and not being able to sit and think about your thoughts.

It is best when you begin an enlightened meditation to start with a calm body and mind. If you're more at ease engaging in the guided meditation and the more comfortable your body and mind are the process, the more open and relaxed your mind will be to the influence of the person who is narrating. The guided meditation process is in manner a type of visualisation. Many studies have proven the effectiveness of visualization. Professional athletes who envision themselves performing well at their chosen sport have been proven to see improvements in their capabilities and performance compared to those who do not think about their performance in sports. People who suffer from strokes and suffer from loss of function in the affected limb because of brain damage are able to build the neural pathway, stop any further damage to the brain and restore function through visualizing the movement of their part of the limb.

The brain does not have the ability to discern between actual and imagined situations. The body, too, can not differentiate between the anxiety that comes from running away from a bear attack and enduring a long working day. The brain is not able to classify events as genuine or fake. It responds in the same way to all. If you go through an hypnotic guided meditation the brain reacts like it was an actual experience. That's why guided meditation and hypnosis are able to be extremely powerful and change your life and ways of thinking in a variety of ways.

Although visualization can be extremely effective it can be, if your mind is blurred and you are having difficulty time focus or concentration when you are doing a visualization, without guidance can be difficult. It's why you should consider an audiobook such as this. Utilizing a narration to guide you through a the guided meditation process can help make a huge difference. The best part about an enlightened meditation is that it allows you to experience a journey to an extraordinary place by positive experiences as well as beautiful images which will be truly real for your brain. This will trigger neural pathways that bring about significant changes to your lifestyle and mind as well as clearing certain "debris" that cause brain fog.

Imagine your brain as an electronic hard drive. There are files and data that are stored in your computer and this is what is the computer's data which is accessible to you. More information you save on your hard drive the more data you are able to access. The caveat is any information you upload to your hard drive is the only data that you will get from it.

As an example, if were taught as a kid that you weren't a good musician, you could save that info in the memory in your head. In and out the mind will affirm that you're not a singer to be reckoned with However, this happens at a sub-conscious level and you're unaware about the "program" that is running on in the background even though it affects and influences your behaviour and how you think about your self. As you get old enough, when someone requests that you sing you won't think about it. You just do the request and simply decline saying that you're an unworthy singer.

It is interesting to note the fact that this idea isn't simply stored in your mind however, it is also a part of your cellular biological. The brain is able to create a route to the information in order and responds to it whenever it is called upon. This happens through neural pathways, but also via unconscious actions that are triggered by your surroundings.

This may sound a bit scary and scary, but what it really implies is that you're not a slave to your genes and you are not bound to become a dependent on your thoughts or past experiences, however you can alter your life as well as your body and your thoughts by altering the data you store on your hard drive. It is possible to alter your life in a way that is cellular by altering the way you think.

There is a possibility that you're familiar with constant confusion. Perhaps you're used to the endless thoughts of stress that plague your mind which contributes to the genesis the mental fog that you are experiencing initially. However, the scientific evidence of visualization proves there's no limit on human capacity to adapt and adapt. Therefore, there's no reason for you to remain in the cloud. It is possible to guide your mind towards clarity and focusing. Beyond that you are able to guide your mind to be empowered throughout your life, by changing the data that is stored in your brain.

The stories that you've repeatedly told yourself for long periods of time isn't easy However, it will take time. If you're persistent and persistent, your old stories gradually become less common as will the more positive and new tales you create for yourself. Just be constant in "rewriting" your messages. There is a need in order to develop the new pathways that connect with your mind and your body. This is the reason why meditation guided is extremely beneficial for physical as well as mental wellbeing.

I would like to emphasize the value of meditation guided so that you don't buy the book and then let it be in the library. I would like you to be that you are compelled to implement this book and practice frequently. To further convince you the advantages of the practice, and to convince you to continue with it Here are additional benefits of guided meditation:

Improving overall well-being and immunity

Reducing the feeling the pain, and also reducing inflammation of the cellular layer.

Increasing your levels of happiness, and increasing your mood.

Reducing anxiety and depression

Reduce stress levels and stress response

Enhancing social interactions and connections by increasing emotional intelligence

Strengthening the cortical region of the brain involved in concentration, which increases your capacity to stay focused and concentrate

Enhancing productivity

Helps to improve memory

Inspiring "outside the box" ingenuity

Allowing for deeper reflection

Increasing your capacity to manage your thoughts and actions

That's it. You are in the right spot. It's time to have the chance to connect with your unconscious, where data plays out on and off throughout the day, and redirect that energy to things that are positive. It's time to provide your brain a fresh sensation through images, sounds or even emotions that you can keep and reinforcing. The time is now to break away from thinking about the past or into the future instead, you will be able to tap in to the present.

With the help of guided meditation, you'll take a huge step toward improving your overall health by opening up your brain and getting rid of the brain fog that hinders the ability of living an active and fulfilling life. This is similar to practicing good hygiene. It's like taking a bath to refresh your mind. According to Indian spiritual coach Sri Sri Ravi Shankar states,

"The value of our lives is based upon the condition of our thoughts." It's time to clean and purify your mind in order to enjoy a more fulfilling living.

A Guide for Meditation

If you've mastered the benefits of meditation and mindfulness, you're ready to begin the journey and begin to learn "how do it". It's great to know that like I said, there are many different forms of mindfulness, as well as various kinds of mindfulness practice. So, get out from your mind the notion that there's only a single "right" method of meditation. If you can incorporate awareness into your day whenever you are aware or being in your surroundings, or you let your mind imagine a positive scenario then you're practicing meditation.

If you're driving for instance, when your mind wandering, without paying attention to the road ahead of you, it is possible to be aware of bringing your focus back to the car you are driving along the road. You can focus on the sound of vehicles honking at your car, the image that appears on your windshield of the highway passing under your vehicle as well as the feel of the rough, sand-like gravel that covers the roadway. When you're taking a stroll or walking, it is possible to focus your attention on the sound of birds singing in the distance, or other details that are sensory to the surroundings. If you're angry over an unfinished phone call finished and you can't get rid of your thoughts about the call then you could shift your focus to the breath and concentrate your attention on the sensation and experience of breathing in and out. You can also do mindfulness meditation and exercise at every time and at any location.

When it comes to more formalized meditation routine, which means setting aside time to relax in a space free from all distractions external to it, in a state of complete concentration on meditative There are a few tips for getting the most benefit out of this practice, and which we'll go through in this section. If you feel that these guidelines to be too unrealistic or unsuitable for you Do not get bogged about having to be unable to perform anything. Here are some suggestions you can be more successful that you are able to pick among based on what's most suitable best for you. The idea is not intended to become the only rule that dictates what you should do. Explore the options and see the best that works for you and let the rest go. When you've figured it out, or after you've thought you've found the answer, you need to be open. Whatever works today could not work for you in the future. However, remember that the practice of meditation can be enjoyable and easy to do.

One of the biggest problems in meditation is that people tend to overcomplicate the procedure making it seem more complicated than it really truly. It's actually quite easy. When your schedule is a mess, and you're required to shut down and reboot, you do not have to do much to help make this occur, as you already have everything you require.

Chapter 10: First Thing You Require Is A Space To Be Seated

When it comes to seated meditation It is essential to understand that seated does not need to be with your legs crossed on the ground, particularly when it doesn't feel comfortable for you. It is possible to find sitting straight in a chair that has an back that is more comfortable, which is less stressful on your back. If you decide to lie down then you might want to do it with cushions to help make it less uncomfortable for your body. It is also the most popular method of meditate and is what you typically encounter when you meditate.

The majority of meditation cushions are cushioned and round or square cushions which are sturdy and lift your body up just a couple of inches above the floor. This support can help maintain your upper body in a straight position but still at ease.

Additionally, it can relieve tension off knees, regardless of the way you sit upon it. The advantage of using an exercise cushion versus the chair is that it makes you much more pressured to keep your posture straight and alert and alert. However, with a seat If you're not cautious it is possible to slump and round your back since the rear of the chair provides an artificial cushion for your back.

If you don't own or are looking for a or a specific meditation cushion, then you can utilize a cushion that is firm or even sit on the couch or in your mattress. However, if you're sitting down while contemplating, it's more comfortable if you're not in a place that's too soft and accommodating. If you're looking for a different alternative, consider an exercise bench. The benches that are made for meditation are little lower than your typical chair and take the strain of your feet off. Additionally, they do not come with a back that encourages users to sit more upright in a chair, similar to cushions. This can be a suitable option for you in case you feel that a cushion will not be comfortable, and you feel that you are losing your focus in the standard chair.

If you're not engaging in an enlightened meditation, the next thing you'll require is a timer. Of course, you don't want to be constantly checking your clock to check the time you're within or outside of the time you've set to meditate. It will surely pull away from what you're trying to focus your thoughts on, and ruin the point of the practice of meditation. Instead, you can create a timer that will chime to signal that it's time to stop the meditation. The easiest method to do this is by using the alarm feature or timer function within your mobile.

However, if you plan to make use of your smartphone for this purpose, I would suggest first eliminating your notifications, and then setting it to airplane mode throughout the practice. In this way you're not tempted to answer any message you receive when you check the phone to set a duration for the session as well as you'll be protected by calls, messages and other notifications which could trigger sounds or vibrate when you're doing your meditation.

You don't want something to distract you from the enjoyment from your journey. In the event that your mobile is in plane mode, that unconscious section of your brain which is waiting for a possible message could be at peace knowing it is impossible for anyone to get in touch with you at the time therefore there's no one you're leaving out or not answering to. If you're looking to expand slightly beyond your basic options, use a meditation app with additional functions which track your practice in meditation or let you know the number of people in the globe are practicing meditation alongside you during that time in order to make sure you're never isolated.

After you've put your tools set, you're set to begin. When you are seated and sit down, you might be thinking about where you're supposed to place yourself. What is the best way to arrange your legs? What do you need to use your arms for? What do you need to do with your hands? When you first lie down, you should ensure that you keep your spine straight. It is the most crucial factor. If you're sitting in a chair that has an backrest, attempt to move the back, making sure that your spine rests against the rear of the chair, and the straightest you are able to be. If you're sitting on a cushion or do not have back support it's still necessary to keep your spine straight as you can. Standing up straight helps you breathe better and more deeply and keeps you focused.

Once you have a clear idea of how your back and spine ought to be doing it is time to consider a few typical positions for your legs. If you're sitting on a meditation cushion, or perhaps a bench, you might find it more convenient to cross your legs. This is the most commonly used approach. Certain people will take it one step further and twist their legs like pretzels to create what's described as a lotus pose in terms of yoga. The second most popular method is to rest your legs. Therefore, when you are in sitting kneeling on the ground then you can place your buttocks upon the rear of your feet. If none of these are suitable for you, it is possible to sit on your feet with legs to the side, and in a straight position. If you're at a desk or sitting on couch or bed You can try the same positions mentioned above as well as sitting while your feet are lying flat on the ground.

The most important thing is to select a place that is comfortable for your legs and back which is comfortable for you and remains comfortable. It will not be distractions throughout the time however, it will help you to remain active. It may require some trials and errors. You may not be aware that sitting with your legs crossed is a good choice initially, but may begin to cause discomfort with time. The next time you'll be able that you should try another pose initially. Be willing to try different things and adjust as you go. The more relaxed you feel and more relaxed, the better meditation experience you'll enjoy.

It's the same for your hands. Do what feels comfortable and normal to you. Take what you are able to sustain for an extended time. The fingers upon your knees. This is the classic "mudra," which looks like it's "okay" hand signal by pressing your forefinger against your thumb and the rest of your fingers are spread out. It's like resting your hands on the legs or knees with your palms open and in the direction of upwards or downwards. palms with the down side facing up.

If you are unsure of what you can do with your eyes, it is possible to keep them closed or open. If your eyes are open, ensure that you close your eyes and keep your eyes gentle. If you have your eyes open this can help draw your eyes down closer, instead of gazing upwards and away. It will not just make you more comfortable and reduce tension for the eyes and your face It will aid in opening your chest and allow you to have an open path to your breathing.

If you test this method and find that the posture is not comfortable for your neck, or the breathing patterns, alter it however you're able to. Eyes open may cause distraction for some and it's recommended that you shut your eyes in order to be more relaxed and enjoy the entire feeling. It's likely to help you to shut out external distracting thoughts and concentrate on the words being told by the speaker during the practice. If you are able to keep closed your eyes, you can tuck the chin towards your chest just a bit. Your goal is to find an area that opens the chest, allowing the air to flow freely.

When you've settled into a relaxed and centered place, it's time to shift from prepping the body for exercise to making preparations for your brain. It's time to narrow your attention. In the course of your day, your thoughts are continuously focusing on your smartphone, news, your work, emails messages, messages, your daily to-do lists, or every other task or obligation and creating an illusion that you're thinking of a thousand things simultaneously, making your mind feel as if it's racing. When you meditate, you're trying to focus your mental focus to a specific target and then try to stay at that spot for a long period of time.

It's straightforward to do However, it becomes more difficult to say when you actually do it because your brain is not accustomed to this. Distractions and stresses of life continually are a constant threat to your brain, pushing it back into the past or into the future, instead of helping it remain within the present. The mind is bound wander and this occurs to the even best-trained meditation practitioners. In the event of this happening the best thing to do is slowly bring your focus back to what you're doing. It's the art of meditation: the continuous focusing and the training of your brain to return to the current time. There will be days that feel more relaxed while others will be much more effort. Whatever happens, you must be gentle and compassionate to yourself. If you become too angry to keep going You'll give up and you won't enjoy the rewards.

That being said and as a final note, these guidelines can differ slightly based upon whether you're performing a walking or seated meditation. This book contains both of them as well, so based the kind of meditation you're practicing change what you're performing with your position and posture, your body and gaze based on what's appropriate to the kind of meditation you're doing during this time.

What To Do When It Gets Difficult

However experienced an individual is in meditation, they will encounter common difficulties, obstacles and misperceptions which need to be dealt with. In this article we'll look at some of them as well as some strategies you can employ to overcome the obstacles and become an effective meditation master.

In the event of a difficulty or challenge in the practice of meditation (or or simply living daily life) Many individuals, particularly those who have no experience, quit. However, obstacles are not uncommon and are actually an essential aspect of meditation. When you face the challenges to train your mind to maintain focus and keep it there to remain capable of overcoming external and internal influencers in your daily day-to-day life.

Every day there will be fluctuations and ups and downs, as well as periods of relaxation and tension. It is, unfortunately, simpler and easier to concentrate on the negative instead of the positive. What you can gain from the past can form you and help your development, and turn your negative experience into something positive experience, if you accept it as an opportunity to learn. It can be difficult but it is much more easily to say than do.

It's also a fantastic method for daily life and it can be applied to your mindfulness and meditation practices as well. There will moments when you're secure, while other times you feel...not at all at ease. At times it can be a struggle. In those moments when you're struggling, instead of becoming discouraged and give up, you'll be able to find out what works and isn't working, and use it in the future sessions of meditation as well as your mindfulness practices.

The obstacles and challenges to mindfulness and MeditationHere are some typical challenges as well with some tips for helping you tackle these challenges and gain knowledge from the experience. It is likely that some of these suggestions will help you in and out of your yoga mat. When you are listening take a step back, open your mind and contemplate ways that you could apply these ideas to everyday life too.

It's a challenge to be mindful. Being aware can feel like an constant, continuous effort. While it may seem easy, it's as though you're constantly working efforts to keep your thoughts where it should be. Concentrating your thoughts on something happening right now can be a gruelling task. Your thoughts are all over moving around and the effort that you make to get attention to what's happening around your eyes is exhausting and seems futile. It seems like it will continue to be this way being present and aware is nearly impossible to maintain.

The advice is that, like everything else that you do, the more you work at it, the better. That means that in first, this may be exhausting and difficult, but as you gain concentration "endurance," the easier it gets. If you're feeling hopeless and helpless in a chaotic environment, getting your mind into the present can give you calm and peace. Mindfulness is a way to find way to ease stress, and not its cause. If you can engage in mindfulness at times that are easy, the simpler to be able to apply it in times that are tough and you'll need this skill for the most.

The challenge is that distractions constantly pull you out of the present. Each time you attempt to keep your thoughts on what's going on in this moment it is interrupted by something else that creates a challenge or even impossible to remain present in the moment. It's like the obstacles and distractions which didn't have any prior existence were suddenly created to make it more difficult for your mind to remain present in the moment which is why you've chosen to take a moment of meditation.

A suggestion: It might be that you feel there are more distractions popping up as opposed to before, but this is likely because you're now more attentive to your thoughts and cognizant of your surroundings. As you meditate, distractions could seem to suddenly "pop out." It might be external distractions, such as the sounds of lawnmowers and the buzz of a fridge or even voices from the room next to you. It could also be inner distractions like sudden recalling specific life issues and drama in relationships, or what you did not complete yesterday, or the negative thoughts that is bubbling up from your past. A lot of this internal and external noise is all the time and is affecting your brain, and you're unaware of it.

The better you are in focusing your thoughts more focused you are, the less significant the distractions become. However, they won't disappear. And you shouldn't expect them to. These distractions provide a great occasion to work on control of your mind. If there were no distractions, how do you improve your concentration? As humans and distractions are likely to occur when they seem to be the least appropriate occasions. It's normal. If framed and utilized correctly, these moments can enhance your mindfulness and meditation practice and allow you to more easily tune into yourself.

The challenge: How long do you think this will be? You've been contemplating for several weeks and are tired of hearing everyone tell you this is an ongoing process. It's going on for a long time, and you're still not seeing any improvement. The process feels tedious and time-consuming, but you don't even see any tangible benefits.

Tips: Remember that it's not the destination that's the primary focus, but the way. If you are tempted to look at the world through a creepy lens, try thinking about what the end goal is for all living things--death. It is the ultimate goal for all living creatures regardless of who or what you're. If you're waiting for something to happen in order to live your life to the fullest, you're wasting your time of the process. Try to be grateful for the time and things that you are currently enjoying. Concentrate on what's going well instead of what's apparent to be happening.

This can help transform your view that stagnation is a sign of awe. From the place where advancement and growth can happen quickly and at the right time. Through your journey of meditation You will experience micro victories that feel great and will give you an opportunity to improve your skills. In time they will build up in your mind, so take them all in and appreciate them at the time. Find a way to feel grateful, even when life doesn't seem to go your way. Keep in mind what the ultimate goal of your life. Don't let your life get in the way. Have fun!

The challenge: You're frustrated. You've attempted to "enjoy the journey" as well as "enjoy the ride" But now more time is gone but your mind is constantly wandering about aimlessly every time you sit down to think. It's time to end at this time as it's being an inefficient use of your time. You've devoted time and energy to this endeavor, and you really tried it and you're not seeing any results out of it. The time has come to time to "throw into the fire."

Tips: At times during any significant and meaningful journey it is easy to quit. Any worthwhile endeavor will experience moments of uncertainty, anxiety as well as anger. The thing you are trying to do is new that is significant and extremely challenging. Thus, the feelings of doubt anxiety, fear and anger can be not just commonplace and normal, they are also expected. These could be an indication that you're in the right direction towards something worthwhile. It is crucial to recognize that these emotions can be temporary. These feelings will fade away.

If you are able to overcome these obstacles, you'll find yourself enjoying things that are to come. You will often find the feelings of anger and anxiety that cause you to let it go will lead you to an important improvement. The times when you're confronted are those when the breakthrough and clarity take place. Keep in mind that even if you're looking to quit it is because you are on the way to something amazing. Keep in mind that, even when you're at a crossroads If you persevere and keep going, you'll enjoy the happiness and growth to come out at hand.

If these seemingly negative thoughts occur, rather than being able to let them make you feel like stopping, let these feelings to motivate your spirit and remind your to continue. Another lesson to learn should be learned through meditation, you are able to implement it in the course of your life. And you'll be grateful to have done so.

Problem: When you start to think about your thoughts and observe the thoughts and feelings that go on inside it the feeling of attachment to emotions or situations develops. It's easy to get caught up in thoughts you'd like to have in the future or recalling incidents from the past. It becomes difficult for you to stay fully present.

Recommendation: As previously mentioned this happens frequently. Everybody, including those with the highest level of experience in mindfulness and meditation practitioners, face difficulties in their daily practice of staying conscious. Non-attachment and letting the world be as they are useful in these situations but it's another ability that will help you not just during the meditation practice, but throughout your the world of.

Aim: The worst spot you'd want to be at this time. Indeed, you'd prefer to be anywhere else than within the present situation that the one you're within. The problem isn't that it's hard to concentrate on anything, however the only thing that your brain is flooded with are scary, painful emotional, heartbreaking, and negative things that you have experienced in the past, or worries concerning the future. You're thinking dark thoughts and it is difficult to think about any other thing. Your thought of remaining there is a sigh of misery and insufferable.

Suggestion: The hard times come for everyone. Nobody's life is flawless And we all go through stress to a certain degree. This is a problem that affects certain people, and affects certain individuals more so than other. Furthermore there are people who are more optimistic or negative or are more optimistic or negative than other people and the place they are in the middle of their temperamental tendencies can have a major difference in how they cope with through, deal with, and go through the life's inevitable challenges. A few people, unfortunately, are quick to succumb to their negative thoughts, which is the inner monster in their heads that nobody else is able to see or hear other than their own.

Instead of trying to fight the issue, mindfulness teachers are encouraging you to accept your present moment in its entirety. Be open to whatever happens as the suppressed state doesn't eliminate it completely It just takes the issue from your mind yet its very presence has a direct impact on every aspect of your life and the way that you present yourself within your daily life. This approach helps you achieve inner peace and also gives you the valuable ability to remain grounded and centered whatever the circumstance.

Problem: It is impossible to think! It's impossible to unwind your thoughts and be able to concentrate on your meditation. The mind is always wandering and your inner dialogue is constantly nagging you over something, and your mind is begging to get rid of everything except clearing out.

A suggestion: Your brain is an active place. If this were a real space to visit, it is Grand Central Station in New York City during the peak of rush hour. The world is always moving in a circular motion, and the signals are constantly changing. Your mind is always considering, thinking about or decoding things. Imagine your intention during meditation is not clearing the mind instead, but to calm them and do not let them to hinder your ability to relax. Focus on your goal.

With the guided meditation, it's somewhat easier as you've got something concrete that you can direct your attention towards. Focus on the words and let them form pictures and imagery that fill your head. If it isn't working for you concentrate on breathing for a while. Consider the amount of time that it takes to breathe in, and then the time it takes to exhale. Your chest will be changing direction with each breath. Be aware of the cool air that it enters your nose and the warm air which escapes your nostrils as you exhale. Let yourself sink into a rhythm that is natural to the breath and then be aware of the breath.

Problem: This is all nice and well, and I'm sure that it is beneficial for a few people, and will improve my life in the future, but who has time to spend time doing this? It's not your time to sit for 30 minutes each day to get your head clear. It's not even fifteen minutes. Not even 5 minutes. There's a job and family members, as well as relationships and a household to keep.

Each day is full of activity starting from the time you wake up until the head rests on your bed at night. You attempt to make an amount of time for meditation However, you're always faced with some thing "more urgent" which pops out that requires attention such as dishes or laundry, a phone call, bathroom breaks and filling up the water bottle, making your outfits ready for the day ahead all the time. There isn't time to meditate because...life.

A suggestion: There's an unwritten rule that financial advisors advise when it comes down to saving money for retirement Do not invest cash on any item until you've paid your own first. This same principle applies to meditation practices. Prior to committing yourself to any activity (or any other person) during the daytime, be attentive to your own needs first. It is not necessary to spend to spend a great deal of time. A minimum of 30 minutes is ideal if you've got time, however 5, 15, and sometimes even two is helpful to improve your mental well-being and clearing your brain of any fog, so that your mind is able to be more efficient and effective in completing the things you have you have to complete. Consistency is the key to success and doing it each throughout the day is ideal.

A few minutes each day are better for your mind than an hour or so once per week. It's not the sort of thing that allows you to skipping it, or be inconsistent or not consider it a serious endeavor and then "make more up for the missing time" by making it a part of your routine. Be consistent throughout time results in the greatest psychological benefits. There's also an added advantage of gaining discipline and willpower which can improve your performance in any other aspect of your day-to-day life.

In case you believe you're lacking time to do it, consider putting things in the context of your goals and prioritizations. Half an hour of meditative time each day might seem as a huge commitment to undertake however, consider asking yourself...were you planning to scroll through your social media accounts for at least an hour? Are you planning to watch the latest episode of a TV show this morning? With under the time you need to view one episode, you could safeguard and maintain your mental wellbeing.

In the case of meditative It can be difficult to get yourself settled and start. Actually, as with almost all things, this is what's the toughest part: starting. Your brain is constantly shouting at you the reasons you shouldn't or shouldn't. When you finally get started it will be evident that you're not ready for this experience to be over.

It is likely that the more time you spend meditating and practice it, the more you'll desire to do it, and you'll like it over other things. Therefore, instead of drowning your brain with mindless activities You will do something beneficial to your brain. You may be enjoying it. Soon you'll find you'll be able to feel more and less boring entertainment and begin to favor meditation instead.

Each meditation within this audiobook have a time-bound length. You aren't able to fit in a five or ten minute time-saver if you're pressed for time as you would when you're contemplating on your own, without any guideline.

It is worth taking time to take the time to utilize these guided exercises every day is the best however, when you are in an time need, you can decide to sit and shut your eyes and be silent for 5 or 10 minutes, instead of not doing anything at all.

Like any other routine you're trying to begin, it may be easier to stick with it by making it part of your routine and pick a fixed time and day when you do it. So, you'll eliminate the uncertainty, the thought process of deciding on the time and where, as well as dissuading yourself from it. Just show to work. Everyday. The same time. Same location. Whatever.

Test: You don't notice any images of swirling colors or shining lights while you meditate. Perhaps you're seeing the things mentioned above, and they're making you feel a little anxious. It's not as if you're floating in the skies, interacting with God with the tang of light all around your. Perhaps you are however, and you're freaking out. Certain people would like to go through these experiences, but others don't. Many people expect this type of experience but it doesn't take place for them. On the other hand, other people don't anticipate this type of thing, but this happens to them. It doesn't matter which the experience can be unpleasant.

The suggestion is that seeing these kinds of things when you meditate does not necessarily suggest that you're a skilled or a meditator. If you don't see them, it doesn't mean that you're doing something wrong. Meditation practitioners are amazing who are able to focus their minds with incredible clarity and a sharpness that has never experienced light, color, or even visions. The focus isn't on getting some awesome response from within your eyelids instead, it's about staying concentrated on the thing you've decided to concentrate on, for example your words during an enlightened meditation.

Chapter 11: Guided Visualization A Walk Through The Forest

Select your ideal location. You can choose to lay down or sit in a reclined position.

If you've decided to lay down or sit ensure that you're at ease, yet not in a place where you are more likely to drift off. It takes a while to relax into the place you prefer. PAUSE 40 SECONDS. If you're not already doing it shut your eyes and make sure that your lips are closed by only allowing your lips be gently in contact. Let go of any tension that is in your face...Relax every muscle that is in your face. From the highest point of your forehead up to your chin...PAUSE for 40 seconds. Let gravity take some of the physical strain off of your body. The surface below you to take on the responsibility of supporting your body. Your body will melt the ground beneath and let the mass of your body to push against the chair, the mattress, the floor and the earth. .... PAUSE 30 SECONDS.

Pay attention to the speed of your breathing. Be aware of the natural pattern of your breathing. PAUSE 30 SECONDS. Are you feeling your breathing hurried? Exasperated? Slow? Tired? PAUSE 40 SECONDS. Take a deliberate, lengthy, slow, deeply breath...and release it at the slowest pace you could, extending the exhale until each piece of oxygen has been taken out of your lungs...PAUSE 20 secs. Repeat this exercise one more time taking a deep breath, inhaling slow, mindfully ....and taking out your breath even slowly, more carefully. PAUSE 25 SECONDS. Relax and allow the slower breathing to gradually slow down the heart rate...One additional time...deep and slow inhale...and exhale long. exhale...PAUSE 25 secs. Then, continue to breathe at a comfortable pace, and allow the stillness to take over your body. Pay attention to the speed of the breath for just a few moments...PAUSE at the end of 1 min.

We're now ready to start our journey. PAUSE 5 SECONDS. The meadow is vast grassy meadow...The thick grass in the meadow is lit by the sun. The light has a warm, soothing feel to the skin. Relaxing in the comforting sensation of warmth from the sun, you gently tilt your head towards the sun, and invite it to shine its light onto your face. It is a good time to look at the sun and to be grateful for its beauty, and appreciate the power it has. It's the primary lighting source all over the world, as well as for other planets that are not our home. It's the vital source of energy for all living things...humans as well as animals and even plants. With each passing second of the sun shining upon your face, it sucks in ever more of its life force into you...PAUSE for 15 seconds.

While your eyes are tilted toward the sun, you find that there aren't clouds visible in the blue sky over you. The colors are so vivid that it draws you in. PAUSE 10 SECONDS. Then you are enthralled by the beauty at the gorgeous blue sky for 7 SECONDS...until it is time to remind yourself of the fact that you're on an open meadow as you can feel the lush grass gently touching your legs. The sudden realization of your legs brings the attention of your feet which are not covered, and allows you to feel cool soil beneath your feet, as well as the soft, moist soil forming itself between your feet. PAUSE 15 SECONDS.

The area in front of you is a vast wooded area. Like the grass that you're standing in is dancing and moves by the soft breeze just like the branches and leaves the trees that are in front of you...as they twist and turn in a circle creating a buzzing sound that will bring a soft smiling smile on your face. The forest's sound ahead of you is enhanced by the varying sounds of the creatures that live in it...the scampers...the chirps...the howls...the sound of coos... PAUSE 1 MINUTE. You see a trail directly in front of you which takes you into the forests. As you walk toward the forest. Every time your foot is placed over another, you notice yourself becoming more comfortable. PAUSE 45 SECONDS.

Be aware of your feet when you walk through this trail. The variety of temperatures and textures of the moss and soil and fallen leaves that line the trail are an enjoyable treat for your feet. The soil is warm and soft due to exposure to sun. The moss is cool, and yet covered with small droplets of morning dew. The leaves are crisp and dry as they shatter and crack every time you step on them. Your only thought in you mind is the wonderful it is to be outdoors with such an amazing view. Unwilling to let it end and continue walking the path...PAUSE for 1 minute. Now you are in the woods. The sounds you heard earlier are getting louder. You can now observe the creatures that were producing the noises you heard a couple of minutes ago, while walking through the meadow. It's a good idea to look around for a few tiny, bright red birds flying in a group in a manner that appears to be playing with each other. It's clear that there's activity within the nearby bushes. Within a couple of minutes the squirrel flies off into the forest, then continues to run ahead of you into the forest seeking food. The wildlife surrounding you, their behaviors as well as the way they interact and their movements, as well as their sounds...PAUSE for 90 seconds.

The air is different. The temperature is cooler because of the denseness of the forests However, occasionally the sun appears through the foliage of the trees, causing sparks of warmth and creates shadows and shapes upon the surface you're traversing. It's a perfect temperature and not too hot but not too cold. ....PAUSE 40 seconds.

It is a good idea to take a breath, breathing in the air from the forest. While you breathe the same, your nose fills with the fragrance of the forest, as its breath makes its way into the lung. Then you breathe in, dissolving the atmosphere and all your worries and anxieties simultaneously at the at the same time. Each time you breathe in you are able to feel a sense of rejuvination, and a sense of refreshment. Every time you breathe out, it feels more peaceful and calm. PAUSE 90 SECONDS.

The trail that took you to the woods goes on. The curiosity of your heart drives you to walk on and discover what it will lead you to. Your muscles relax as you take each step. Your body is free of tension after each breath. The arms move effortlessly in perfect harmony when you move. They're loose and relaxed. Your back is comfortable and straight...PAUSE for 10 seconds.

The trail begins to climb however it's accessible to walk... While you progress you realize that the earth changes. The ground is changing...not just the gradual slope and slope, but the ground that was soil, moss, or leaves has changed into soft stones. The stones are held by your feet while walking, and while you travel down the road, each step feels like a appreciated massage to the sole toes. PAUSE 10 SECONDS. The breeze is still passing through the trees, helping to keep you cool as well as comfy. A certain aspect of the shade provided by trees can make you feel calm, as if it's going to remain in order. PAUSE 15 SECONDS. The greenery changes and shifts and gradually getting more vivid while you progress on the hill. It is possible to see a variety of shades of green in the trees...some are dark and deep, but others appear light and look almost translucent. However, they all work with each other to create a stunning landscape surrounding your.

While focusing on the colors that leaves appear to be, glance at the bark that the tree has... The various colors...and textures...Some trunks appear glossy and smooth, while other trunks are dark and rough. The bark's colors are wildly different from one tree to next one, varying higher than the hue of bark could. It's been a while since you've seen such various shades of bark...shades of orange, brown, peach...all so different, yet equally stunning. Pay attention to the fine details of the trees as you walk. PAUSE 1 MINUTE.

The trail begins to climb downhill, until there is a tiny stream that is babbling along the trail, and continues downwards. It is located on a huge, flat rock right adjacent to the stream. It's perfectly positioned so as to invite the user to lay down and take in the sound of the river when it runs over rocks and other stones and sticks to its course. It's time to stop your walk and you sit down on the rock and observe the temperature and how it feels beneath your body. PAUSE 45 SECONDS. Once you've settled down on the rocks, slip your feet into the cool, fresh and crystal clear water let it flow through your feet and tuck on your heels. PAUSE 15 SECONDS. As you get more comfortable lying down on the rocks, resting your feet in the stream, as the sun shines upon your face. The light air smacks against your skin and the sweet scent of the fresh forest fresh air fills your nose. PAUSE 1 MINUTE. You feel calm, grounded, and connected, you are able to take into everything surrounding you...every sensation it evokes and every feeling it evokes...as your brain becomes relaxed and clear. STOP 2 MINUTES.A quiet, but abrupt noise catches your attention and prompts you to get down on the rocks. Just across the way is an animal drinking from the stream. The deer raises her head, and stares at you. She's relaxed and isn't worried, nor do you. You observe her as she resumes drinking, marveling the ease with which you can see her move. You marvel at how she's serenely in the moment, and has no worries about the future, and no worries regarding the past. She is totally focused on her activities in the present moment. It is important to take note of your observation in order to keep an ongoing reminder to stay relaxed and present as the deer. PAUSE 20 SECONDS. Deer takes one last drinking of water, then goes back to the forest returning to her home and reminding you to go back to your own. PAUSE 7 SECONDS. Slowly restore your focus to your body. Begin by focusing on the feet...Wiggle the toes gently...wiggle the fingers gently...PAUSE 20 secs. When you're ready to open your eyes, slowly and remember that you are able to be back in the woods any time you want or need to. The forest will always be waiting to welcome you, waiting and ready to meet your, restore you and help you relax.

Walking & Movement

There is no need to sit in a secluded spot in order to be meditative. Today, we'll show the point. If you're still not going outside, start walking ....PAUSE for 15 seconds. There is no doubt that exercise has positive effects that extend beyond the physical appearance or well-being. Exercise has been proven to ease stress, clear your mind, increase the flow of thoughts and stimulate imagination. Ironically, exercise may also aid in relaxation. It can also help to promote the release of trapped energies...physical physical, mental, as well as emotional. Therefore, today instead of traditional sitting in silence and solitude We are going to get our bodies moving.

Everyday, everything around us is constantly in motion, and trying to get our attention...The ideal way to stay sane in spite of that reality is to rely on the power of controlling our thoughts to be quiet, calm and peaceful regardless of the constantly moving around us. When you are out and about, this practice will bring you back to real daily life and all the distractions. It will help you train your mind to be calm, focused and focused on the things you decide to pay attention to regardless of what's happening in the world around you. The practice will help the importance of being more attentive of your daily routine and to pay attention to and appreciate every little thing in front of your. If your climate is causing you to feel wind, sun or a chill, getting outdoors, or even getting a fresh breath is enough to be in touch with nature that is among the most effective ways to boost the quality of your life and mental state...

We will now start the prayer...

It is normal to walk ....just walk naturally...PAUSE for 30 SECONDS...notice the speed of your walk...is it fast? ?...is it fast ?...are you moving in a manner that suggests you need to be by a specific time ?...PAUSE for 10 SECONDS...or is it slower ?...is it slow? ?...PAUSE five SECONDS...Take time to look at your pace ....and think about what ideas are influencing your speed ....PAUSE 15 seconds. If you're moving fast...why do you walk in such a hurry? ?...If you're moving slowly...why? Somewhere in between?...Why?...There is no good or bad, no right or wrong. Just observe...and ask yourself...why...PAUSE 60 SECONDS.

While you aren't trying to alter any thing, be aware of how your weight is distributed across your feet while they press down on the ground as they move. Do you feel that the weight is distributed evenly? Is there a particular part of your foot receive greater pressure than other areas? PAUSE 60 SECONDS.

Then, slow your speed a bit. Enjoy the slow speed. Be aware of what the slower pace does to your mood and the thoughts that are circulating in your head. It could be that the slower pace can calm your mind. If you're used to a faster or more fast pace, you could begin to experience anxiety and desire to speed up to get back on track. Be aware of the feelings that arise within your body, and how thoughts pop into your mind. PAUSE 90 SECONDS.

Pay attention to your feet's soles. Be aware of how each part your foot is in contact with the ground while your feet roll every step. Notice how the muscles of your foot relax and contract when you move. Do you notice any part of your foot contracts as you walk, like you were trying to hold the surface? Do you notice that this slower speed affect the way you feel your feet as well as the way you walk are feeling? PAUSE 90 SECONDS.

Spend the time to be aware of the feelings caused by anything you touch. PAUSE 10 SECONDS. Do you have socks on? Do you have the pants? What is the way that the fabric of your footwear, socks or your pants make your feet feel? Do the fabrics of your pants touch the skin, causing it to itch and irritate your ankles? What is the feel of your shoes on your feet? ?...Are they tight on your feet, or does your foot allow for movement inside your footwear? PAUSE 60 SECONDS. Are you wearing closed or open toe footwear? Does that impact how your feet feel? Are your shoes making your feet feel warmer? Are your feet soaked from sweat? If you're wearing open toe footwear, are the conditions altering the temperature of your feet? Are you feeling sun upon the bottom of your shoes? ....a breeze...a cool? PAUSE 70 SECONDS.

Bring your attention up to your legs and bring your attention back to your lower legs. Focus on your shins and calves. Pay attention to your sensations...your clothing...your temperature...the manner in which your muscles relax and relax...PAUSE for 60 seconds. Begin to work your way to your knees, and then your legs on the upper side. Your thighs' muscles are among the most powerful in your body. What do they feel like? How are they acting and alter when you walk? PAUSE 60 SECONDS. What happens to your hips as you walk? How is your pelvis moving? PAUSE 30 SECONDS. What does each part of your lower body function in concert? Be aware of how effortless each component of your lower body understands exactly what needs to be done. Each body part is with perfect harmony, giving you the ability to move. PAUSE 45 SECONDS.

Your attention has been your attention on the lower portion of your body. This is the body part that is doing most of the work when you're walking...or do you? What's happening to your upper body while you stroll? It's your spine...your stomach...your back...the motion of your arms...the motion of your shoulders and chest when you breathe? What do you think of your neck when it holds your head? Do you notice that your head is bowed little, synchronized with your step? Be aware of the upper part of your head. PAUSE 1 MINUTE.

After you've spent the entire time being aware of your body, turn your focus to the outside. It is easy to get caught within our own space within our heads and surrounded by those same thoughts that keep revolving within our minds, until you walk around in blindfolds. Our eyes are closed to world around us. Spend a few minutes observing your surroundings without judgment, not making judgements about the things you see, and making assumptions regarding the things you see...just look around, paying close particular attention to the smallest seeming minor things. PAUSE 2 MINUTES.

Check out the possible sounds you identify...voices engaged in conversation when you stroll by pedestrians in the sidewalk...dogs barking...a plane hovering overhead...horns honking...try to pick up even the most subtle and insignificant of sound. PAUSE 2 MINUTES.

Look around the structure and infrastructure that surrounds you...there was an time where none was in existence. Every thing you see was created and created by humankind...an oft-forgotten reminds us that what we imagine in our heads is what we are able to create the world around us. Pay attention and notice...the walkway that lies under your feet...a bridge that lies in the distance...the surrounding buildings and entice you by their meticulously chosen colours, intriguing shapes and lines shapes...Look at all the objects that man has built and used to build, some useful and some stunning, but some of them both...PAUSE for 2 minutes.

Humanity's creations are amazing, however what nature has created is superior because it occurs with no effort. Humanity must think, make plans, and construct and work to build. Nature is just that. Nature produces beauty and perfection in a matter of seconds. ....Observe the beauty of nature all around you...a tree...a plant...grass...a flower...for in the remaining few moments, marvel at nature's beauty marvel, beauty, and beauty. PAUSE 2 AND A HALF MINUTES.

Finally, take a look at the other people surrounding you...PAUSE 15 secs. Although we're all basically the same on the inside, sharing the same wants, dreams and fears hopes...we are all different from the outside. Be aware of the many variations in the shapes and sizes that our bodies come in...the various ways that we decide to style our clothes as well as our hair to represent us and convey a message to other people about who we really are and the person we wish to be perceived as. PAUSE 10 SECONDS. Be aware of the beauty unique to everyone around you. PAUSE 30 SECONDS.

Try looking deeper...at faces...body language...What are people's expressions say about them? How can their expressions change as you smile? Smile at someone you don't know and observe the impact it has on their expressions. PAUSE 45 SECONDS. In the midst of our own issues that we don't consider what eye contact and a quick smile could do for another person. We aren't able to make connections. There is no way to tell what people we have in common with our loved ones, friends or business partners aren't able to make relationships with due to our failure to invest the time and effort into building a relationship. There is no eye contact, or communicate which means that we don't have the opportunity of being able to receive and give love...Each person you meet is a person with a story, a story that deserves empathy, the kind of compassion we are often unable to offer. We don't realize what the other person is suffering, so we frequently make the wrong assumption that our troubles are more serious than those surrounding us. PAUSE 30 SECONDS.

In bringing this meditation to an end, breathe deeply through and out, and think of the following thought:

Chapter 12: The Sky Of Your Mind

The most frequent anxieties is feeling lonely. The reason is simple. If we're in a room by ourselves, we can't have anyone else around to help us escape the endless chatter inside our minds. One of the most unsettling ways for people to do is just to be alone and think their own thoughts. When the mind is allowed to wander, may be prone to catastrophize, judge, and criticize and even express fear or doubt and even shame. However, when you allow an issue to arise and be released, it is possible to let it go to let it pass or clearing your thoughts, or allowing room for a positive or productive way of thinking. This meditation am taking a step back in order to allow you an opportunity to spend time contemplating your own inner thoughts without distractions and only a little guidance. This may feel uncomfortable, it could be a challenge and even painful, but it's a necessity.

It is important to take a few minutes to settle in a relaxed, comfortable place. Make sure your back is straight and supported if needed. The meditation will start by paying attention to your breathing. Pay attention to your natural breathing while you breathe in and out. PAUSE 40 SECONDS. Then, you can begin to increase the depth of the breath by breathing in slow and deep, and then fully exhaling all of the air. While doing this relax, let the tension of the muscles in your body to release...PAUSE at 45 seconds.

Switch your focus towards your thoughts. PAUSE 10 SECONDS. Then you may begin to think about self-judgments, things that you would like to change about your life, issues you would like to change concerning yourself...or concerning others...things unfinished that you need to get done, tasks that you think you could be doing differently or better and worries about what's likely to occur in the future...whatever you think about, simply let it upwards similar to bubbles that get bigger and rise towards the highest point. This meditation isn't to stop thinking. It's to watch your thoughts with no attachment and with no judgment. When a thought comes up just let it wander through your mind as clouds that are in the sky. Simply watch it pass as a cloud glides over the sky or like an helium balloon is lifted in the air before floating out into the wind. Take note of it, but do not be attached. PAUSE 5 MINUTES.

Everything is wrong. Everything is right. All that is needed is. PAUSE 2 MINUTES.

Your brain is like the sky that is above you. Its vast clean, unending ....Light is shining onto your world through the sun. The light you receive is wisdom as well as your clarity and positivity. In the course of the day, there are clouds that appear and disappear as thoughts be a blur. Storms can even move in and block the sun for a short time. At times, it might become dark, bleak even. However, this doesn't mean the sun will not be shining. It will return. The sun is blocked until the time. The sky is aware of this, and therefore is not disturbed by a new storm. It is not agitated with the storms. They simply pass by and disappear. The sky does not represent the cause of the storm. Sky isn't cloud. It's just a place to allow clouds through. The same way you're not the thoughts. Your mind is just an area for thoughts to move through. Sky does not have the power to decide what clouds are, just in the same way that you do not need to be able to judge your thoughts. The sky lets clouds move through the grandeur of it. They do not diminish the splendor, grandeur or the transparency that the skies offer. They come and then leave. Sky remains. You should take a moment to be amazed by the amazing and stunning sky in your head is. PAUSE 45 SECONDS.

Be aware of your thoughts. At any time an emotion, thought or image or feeling arises you can allow it to exist and let it go through your mind. PAUSE 6 MINUTES.

When we allow thoughts or emotion to sway our thoughts, we loose connections. When we give the significance of every thoughts that arise and lose our perspective and lose strength and our capacity to manage things the manner they should be dealt with. It's as if clouds have taken over the sky. However, we forget when we do that, it is us who are the sky and not the clouds. The sole function of the sky is provide your thoughts with a place to wander but keep your thoughts calm and quiet. The sky is you rather than the clouds. Being aware, but not being overwhelmed...

PAUSE 5 MINUTES.

As we navigate the day-to-day routine We often do not realize the amount of mental energy is devoted to worry or anxiety. The thoughts are constantly racing through our brains, taking our minds of focus, peace, and joy. Let those thoughts have space today to enter your mind and move through your mind to let go of their influence within your daily life. Let each thought occur without emotional attachment or reacting to it...PAUSE for 5 minutes.

Get a few more deep breaths. PAUSE 30 SECONDS. Refocus your attention back on the hands ....moving them gently...your feet...moving them gently...Take an additional deep breath before slowly exhaling the air via your nostrils. In the process of letting go of this mindfulness practice, be aware that every moment, every idea, is as the cloud. Your mind is like the sky. If you are feeling stuck in the middle of a severe storm and you are unsure if the storm will end, remember that you're the sky, not clouds. If you are feeling overloaded or engulfed within your thoughts, glance towards the sky and allow it to serve as an encouragement to remember that you don't have to become overwhelmed by each thought that comes into your mind. It is enough to let the thoughts drift away like a cloud in sky...You might now be able to open the eyes...

Finding Clarity in Your Breath

A very easy basic, but profound practices for meditation that you can adopt is focusing your attention on breathing. Breathing deeply and in a full, continuous way will not only supply oxygen into your bloodstream and circulates oxygen to the brain, that can aid in removing the fog in your brain and bring mental and physical energy into your entire body. Through this practice, you are going to focus on your breathing rhythm and link it to the idea of purification and release. In the process the body will be restored to equilibrium, returning to the "natural" and peaceful condition of mind.

Now, let's start...

You must ensure that you're in the most comfortable spot to relax. PAUSE 5 SECONDS. This could happen sitting on an chair...a bed...a sofa...just be sure you're sitting at a location that can allow you to be at ease for the length of the practice. PAUSE 5 SECONDS. Relax for a few seconds into your new position. ....PAUSE 5 secs. Set your legs and ....relax and your shoulder ....place them in a manner that feels comfortable to you...PAUSE 15 secs. Close your eyes and take a moment to concentrate on the breath... PAUSE 15 SECONDS. For the next 15 seconds, be aware of your breathing. ....If you are finding it hard to remain focused in your breathing, you can begin taking a count of your breath...Count every second you exhale ....and take note of each second that you exhale. after which, when you take your next breath begin over...just keep breathing and keep counting. PAUSE 30 SECONDS.

While you breathe as you continue to breathe, consider a goal to the meditation. Pick a simple sentence which describes the outcome you'd want to accomplish from the session. This could mean finding your mental clarity, which will make it much easier to resolve a dilemma you've had in your mind...it may be to feel more grounded and connected, so that you are able to bring greater motivation to your relationships...it may be to reenergize and reenergize yourself to be ready for the new coming day ahead...it is entirely up to you...Take the time to tune into how you're thinking and then choose the intention you would like to pursue. PAUSE 30 SECONDS. After you've chosen your goal Repeat it three times to form a kind of mantra for your mind. This will help you to remember it. It will set the stage to the practice. PAUSE 40 SECONDS.

Let go of all thoughts about your goal and return your attention towards your breathing. ....PAUSE 10 secs. Then, we'll commence an alternate nostril breath method that is popular in pranayama yoga as it can help to rejuvenate the body, enhance sleep to help relax the nervous system and regulate body temperature and enhance your mental function...As you keep breathing slowly lift your left hand to your nose. Then utilize your index finger to close your left nostril. Take a slow inhale through your right nostril. when the air enters imagine it moving upwards through your nose, as well as all the way to the bottom of the lungs below. ....When you've finished the inhale, hold your nose shut for a few seconds to stop your breathing. Release the left hand from the left nostril. However, hold the right nostril shut by using your thumb. Take a deep breath out of the left nostril. When all air is gone from your lungs, you can imagine confusion, brain fog or all other mental impurities that are leaving the same way. Repetition this breathing exercise at your own speed. Let me walk you through it once more time. Keep your nose closed to the left with the index finger. breathe through your left nostril, ...pinch the nose shut and then pause for a second and then let the index finger of your left nostril, then breathe out through it, with your thumb still on the inside of your right nostril. Then, you can take the next two minutes to repeat the process. Remember, don't rush. PAUSE 2 MINUTES.

We're going perform the same procedure and reverse the process. This time it is important to close your nose on your right side using your thumb. Breathe in via the left...pinch your nose...then allow your thumb to exhale from the right nostril. Deeply and slowly breathe Repeat this procedure. PAUSE 2 MINUTES.

Take your hands off your nose, and let your hand return to its initial position and rest comfortably. Take a slow inhale throughout both nostrils. ....Feel the breath in your lungs as it fills them.

www.ingramcontent.com/pod-product-compliance
Lightning Source LLC
Chambersburg PA
CBHW070555010526
44118CB00012B/1320